Praise for
Adventures in Physical Therapy—

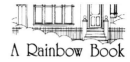

Λ Rainbow Book

Dr. Figueroa shows his goodness and his sensitivity to the human condition as he tells his patients' stories. His steadfastness with them makes us realize we should never 'quit' on our patients and that they should not quit on themselves when life puts obstacles in their way. It makes the reader realize how important we are in our patients' lives, even if it is for a short duration. Physical therapists are often their rock and their hope. We are definitely their greatest cheerleaders. This is a must read for all physical therapists and for anyone who wants to enter a health profession. It is also a must read for anyone experiencing pain. Pain and suffering are often a part of the human condition, and Dr. Figueroa shows how, through hard work and dedication, a better outcome can be achieved. As Dr. Figueroa's former professor and professional colleague, I am so proud of him for his dedication to excellence, for his kindness and caring, and for his openness to helping his fellow human beings.

—Eileen Hamby, DBA, PT

Adventures in Physical Therapy: Stories to Ease the Pain is a book for many readers but will benefit patients and their caregivers, prospective and health career professionals, and others who desire a bit of humor, motivation, and lessons that can be learned through real life stories. The author, Fernando Figueroa, shares some of his adventures that "impacted his life and beliefs," reflecting his success as a highly knowledgeable and compassionate individual contributing to the care of his patients while making friendships along the way. A book to have on your shelf to share with a friend in need!

—Leila J. Darress, PT, MS-HSA,
former program director (1996–2013),
Physical Therapist Assistant Program,
Indian River State College

Praise, continued

Praise, *continued*

Adventures in Physical Therapy was a good read. I like the title because each patient is an adventure—and the challenge. This book has warmth and the depth of friendship that you develop with the patients as they struggle after a surgical adventure, and the nurturing back to health, both mentally and physically.

On the surface it appears to be just a detailed description of the patient's problem, but underneath it's the perseverance, motivation, and experience that brought out the moral fiber and constitution of the individual, and how to help the patient conquer his adversity.

The book details the experiences of a broad spectrum of personalities and problems that are dealt with on a daily basis.

—Frank D. Murphy, M.D.,
Orthopedic Surgeon, Stuart, Florida

Most people dread going to physical therapy. They know broken arms and legs must be moved, muscles must be stretched, and they know it's going to hurt. As a former patient, I have a suggestion: If you need a physical therapist, try to see Fernando Figueroa. He is knowledgeable, intelligent, and totally focused on making his patients better. He also knows how to keep them upbeat while they're doing the hard work of recuperating.

But if you can't see him, buy this book and take it with you to therapy. *Adventures in Physical Therapy: Stories to Ease the Pain* is a charmer of a book. It will make you laugh, make you think, and will teach you something—if you pay attention.

—Sandra J. Robson, author of *False as the Day Is Long*

Adventures in Physical Therapy

Stories to Ease the Pain

Fernando Figueroa,
PT, DPT, Ph.D., Cert. MDT

Rainbow Books, Inc.
F L O R I D A

Library of Congress Cataloging-in-Publication Data

Figueroa, Fernando, 1964-
   Adventures in physical therapy : stories to ease the pain / Fernando Figueroa, PT,
DPT, Ph.D., Cert. MDT.
       pages cm
   ISBN 978-1-56825-185-1 (trade softcover : alk. paper) -- ISBN 978-1-56825-186-8
(epub e-book)
   1. Physical therapy--Anecdotes. I. Title.
   RM701.F44 2015
   615.8'2--dc23

                           2014048135

            Adventures in Physical Therapy: Stories to Ease the Pain
               © 2016 by Fernando Figueroa, PT, DPT, Ph.D., Cert. MDT

               Author's Website: FernandoPhysicalTherapy.com

ISBNs
       Softcover 978-1-56825-185-1
       EPUB e-book 978-1-56825-186-8

Published by
       Rainbow Books, Inc.
       P.O.Box 430
       Highland City, FL 33846-0430
       Telephone (863) 648-4420
       Fax (863) 647-5951
       RBIbooks@aol.com
       RainbowBooksInc.com

Orders
       •   *Wholesale*, contact Rainbow Books, Inc.
       •   *Retail*, contact Rainbow Books, Inc. for your online discount code
       •   *Individuals*, ask your local booksellers to order ISBN 978-1-56825-185-1,
            shop online, or call 1-800-431-1579 (all major card accepted).
       •   *Online*, find your best online hard copy price at AllBookStores.com (search
            for ISBN 978-1-56825-185-1).
       •   *Professional*, bulk-purchase discounts are available to physical therapy or
            medical professionals by contacting the publisher.

            Cover images: iStockPhoto • Author photo: Audra Bell

Disclaimer: The stories in this book are for entertainment purposes only and should not
be used as substitute guidelines for actual physical therapy. Physical therapy routines
are prescribed and are unique to each patient. Names and identifying information have
been changed.

   First Edition 2016 • Written, produced and printed in the United States of America

To my children, Andrea and Christian, who I love with all my heart.

To Audra, my soulmate.

To my family, friends, and especially to my patients, who inspired me to write this book.

CONTENTS

PREFACE

I always thought my first book would be related to physical therapy: either manual therapy or spine biomechanics, or an orthopedic matter, which describes my work and specialization. After twenty-six years' experience, plus the years I was a student, I have chosen to share stories of patients and colleagues. These stories have shaped, in many ways, how I view my life, my clinical practice, and my beliefs.

The idea for this book came to me years ago when I was co-owner at another physical therapy office. One day, when I was working with a patient, I told him a funny story I remembered about another patient in a similar situation. He laughed so much that the painful therapy became less stressful, and he appreciated the distraction. He used it in an optimistic way to control the pain caused by his sessions. After that, he insisted I put all my stories together in one book.

I thought it was a good idea, but as the years passed I was dedicated to finishing my Doctorate in Physical Therapy (DPT) and starting a solo PT practice. Then another patient, with whom I'd used a past patient's story, recommended the same thing to me—that I write a book—and this time I decided to do something about it.

I was very sick the first few years of my life. I was unable to participate with family and friends in many birthdays, parties, and Christmas celebrations because I was always sick in bed or in the recovery process. I suffered with pneumonia several times and survived every single childhood disease you can imagine. My immune system was quite limited, and many times I had to visit the hospital, doctors' offices, and labs for different tests.

My pediatrician, Dr. Saavedra, who I still remember dearly, was the only one who gave hope to my parents, especially my mother. She was the one who went with me to the hospital, along with my grandma, who was a nurse. Dr. Saavedra said, "Leave the child alone. He will be okay by the time he's ten years old," and he was right, because I remember a big change at that age. I began to feel great; I wanted to do everything previously forbidden because of my ailments. I drove my parents crazy when I started to play basketball, soccer, and other sports. I wanted to make up the exercise time I had lost.

Years passed, and I found I enjoyed science more than any other subject. In high school, once a week, we were introduced to different careers. During one particular week we focused on the career objectives for a kinesiologist, or physical therapist. The combination of science and exercises caught my attention and fascinated me. I knew right away that my exposure to the medical world, so young in life, and to sports, which had been taboo for so long, foretold my future path. It was an easy decision to make, and I became a physical therapist at the age of twenty-two.

Physical therapy practice involves very close work with patients in hospitals and nursing homes, as well as home health and outpatient settings, and the process takes several weeks, sometimes longer. In the dynamic healthcare service of PT, practitioners have the chance to develop positive relationships with patients as part of our role as health care providers. As an educator, it is important to instruct and motivate them to perform the proper movement, the proper activity, and to become more independent and safe. Ultimately, we develop a very important aspect of rehabilitation: trust. Once we achieve trust, we can convince patients to follow specific therapeutic exercises, even though they may result in pain.

The stories that follow are real, some of them are quite funny, others very sad. Each has given me a lesson to learn. Names of patients, as well as any identifying information, have been changed to protect patients' identities. I hope you enjoy reading the stories as much as I did writing them.

CHAPTER ONE

The Lady and the Cat

—Fernando Figueroa

I went to help a nice lady who had undergone surgery for a total knee replacement. Rebecca was recovering at home, which is where I started her therapy.

Following the protocols and procedures of her case, I asked Rebecca if she lived alone or if she had family living with her. She told me she still grieved the loss of her husband, who had died the year before.

While she told me about her loss, her cat jumped from corner to corner of her bed, off the bed and back on the bed. I like animals, but the cat would not stop, and I was getting annoyed. I asked her to help me with the cat so I could perform my therapy without interruption.

Rebecca moved the cat and mentioned she had never liked cats. During her married years, she and her husband never had a cat, mainly because of her allergies. Her husband, she said, had always wanted a cat, but he never insisted on getting one because he didn't want to make her sick.

I had to ask her, "Why do you have a cat now?"

She explained how, the day she came back home after her husband's funeral, she was devastated by the feeling of emptiness so common after such a loss. "That very night," Rebecca said, "I woke up to a noise. I couldn't understand what it was but got up and went to the front door to see. The cat was outside. I opened the door and found the cat meowing. I was irritated after being woken up, so I pushed the cat away and went back to sleep."

The following couple of nights, the cat returned, meowing her awake, and again she had to push it away. She was beginning to get tired of the situation.

One morning her daughter came to visit, and Rebecca told her daughter what had happened the previous two nights with the cat. While they talked, she and her daughter opened the garage to look for something stored inside. The cat darted past them, into the garage, and went straight to a corner where a big snake lay coiled. Both the mother and daughter were shocked at the situation, especially when the cat came to them with the snake in its mouth. The cat placed the now-dead snake in front them, as if saying, "Well, I am here to help!"

Obviously, she couldn't refuse that kind of help, and she immediately adopted the cat. Her biggest surprise was she never had any allergies related to the cat.

I told her the cat was sent by her husband to take care of her.

I had an opportunity to meet Rebecca some time later, after she suffered a stroke that afflicted her with a severe paralysis on one side of her body. Because of her limitations, she hired a private aide to help her with her basic activities of daily living.

One night her cat saved her again. One of her aides abandoned Rebecca during the night, leaving her asleep and alone.

Close to 10:30 PM, the cat jumped on her night table and pushed a glass of water onto her. She woke up and called for help, but the aide was not there, and nobody came to help her. Rebecca was alone with her cat but was able to use her phone to notify someone of the situation.

As you can imagine, the cat's actions revealed that a caregiver had taken advantage of Rebecca and her family, and the aide agency very quickly took care of the problem employee.

I am convinced that, in some way, the cat was connected with Rebecca's husband.

Recently, I stopped by to check on Rebecca and learned her cat died after many years with her. I saw a look in her eyes as if she too were saying goodbye. I gave her a kiss on the forehead and left, knowing her time would come soon.

CHAPTER TWO

A Surgeon from the Vietnam War

I worked in Houston, Texas when I was a young physical therapist. During my first week, I was introduced to the entire staff at the hospital. I heard a lot about one very good surgeon, Dr. X, who was a little "special" because of his actions.

On my third day at the hospital, I worked with my boss and another PT in an isolated room with a whirlpool. We were treating a very contagious patient who suffered from an abdominal wound infected with pseudomonas, a contagious bacterium. Our protocol included changing our clothes from top to bottom—similar to performing surgery—and wearing goggles to avoid any contact with the bacteria.

In the middle of the procedure, someone opened the door, and there stood Dr. X, the famous surgeon I had heard about from day one. I was shocked to see him, especially because he was wearing a suit and tie! The patient was very happy to see Dr. X, who donned a glove on one hand to check the patient's wound.

After he examined the wound, he took off his glove, threw it in the garbage can, walked over to the whirlpool (the same whirlpool in which the patient had received treatment), and washed his finger with the water!

My boss introduced me to him, and Dr. X stretched out his hand for a handshake. The problem was, I was so shocked with his poor universal infection precautions that I extended only a gloved hand.

It was natural for him not to care about the health precautions. We couldn't say anything in front of the patient about the incident, but my boss was not surprised by what had happened. He said Dr. X was a great surgeon who had learned the majority of his skills as a physician in the Vietnam War. At some point during the war, he no longer had sanitary equipment to work with. Because he was focused on saving as many lives he could, he got used to not paying attention to handwashing protocols.

The entire whirlpool had been contaminated!

Sometime later, I worked with a patient who had a nasogastric tube placed through her nose and into her stomach by Dr. X after abdominal surgery. She sat in her chair while I washed my hands after my work with her.

When Dr. X entered the room, he said hello to me, and we talked about the patient's condition. He was happy with her progress, he told her, so he decided to remove the tube.

The patient was surprised when she realized Dr. X had decided to do it—right then and there. She was terrified when he said, "Okay, Mrs. Smith, take a deep breath . . ." Before she could say anything, he pulled the tube as if tugging a garden hose, and it came out with all kinds of mucus and fluids attached. He put the tube and its contaminants in the garbage and went to the sink, while telling her everything went fine.

He washed only his fingers!

I still remember her face; she was exhausted from the whole ordeal. The only thing I could tell her was, "You are one step closer to leaving the hospital to go home."

I will always remember Dr. X and his great surgical skills. But most of all I will never forget that he thought just washing only his fingers—not his hands—was sufficient.

CHAPTER THREE

Mark, the Man Who Was in a Coma for Six Years

Mark was very successful businessman and an only child. He and his girlfriend lived in an apartment close to his parents in New Jersey. One stormy day he was driving his car home from work when he decided, due to dark and wet conditions, the highway was his best choice.

He began to have difficulty reaching the highway because the rain poured down so hard the roads quickly filled up with water. As the water began to rise on the roads, Mark had to figure out a way to avoid further problems. He drove through one curve and lost control of his vehicle.

According to the police, his car hydroplaned and ran straight into a tree. The impact was so horrible that when the emergency crew arrived at the scene, they thought Mark was dead.

Luckily, they were able to resuscitate Mark after performing CPR for several minutes. He arrived at the hospital with severe fractures to his right femur, left shoulder, and ribs. But he had a brain injury. He survived several orthopedic surgeries for his femur but was still in a coma.

Several weeks passed, and Mark was sent to another hospital to continue his recovery, but he remained in a coma. His mother and father were by his bedside every time they were allowed. The medical bills were stacking up, and they were given little hope regarding their son.

After a year with no improvement, his family made a decision to move him to another facility. They sold their house in New Jersey and moved to North Carolina so Mark could stay in a less expensive nursing home to help stretch their dwindling money as much as they could. After two years they again ran into a similar situation: dwindling money and hope.

They decided again to sell another property and moved to Florida, where they had relatives to help them. In Florida, they moved Mark to different nursing homes, looking for the most suitable one for them and for their son. His mother had been by his side every day since the accident. She prayed and prayed for God to bring her son back. Talking to her years later, she told me she never lost faith or hope because she knew one day the miracle she had been waiting for would come to fruition. She prayed for six years, two weeks, and three days. (It amazes me even to write this.)

One miraculous day, God fulfilled her request. After many years of no reaction of any kind, Mark finally opened his eyes. He was unable to talk because of the respirator tube in his mouth. The miracle became even more amazing when Mark's vitals signs improved. The respirator was removed, and Mark was able to breathe on his own. His body was full of stiffness, but he had no open sores or any kind of wounds, thanks to the love and care of his parents.

They described his finger as being like a piece of wood (referring to stiffness), which showed how long he had been in a coma. After waiting for so long for Mark's miracle, the family was filled with joy. Even though they knew Mark would eventually wake up, they also knew it was the beginning of a long process.

Mark's speech returned, but he couldn't remember anything: who he was, who his family was, and what had happened before and after the accident. Everything was new to him. His parents tried everything they could to make him understand and to regain his memory. They showed him old pictures to help him remember.

After nearly eight months awake, he was released from the nursing home to start outpatient therapy.

Mark's parents brought him to see me as a new patient in October of 1992. His parents brought him in a special wheelchair that reclined. He was unable to sit up, not only because of the weakness, but because of the stiffness that ebgulfed his whole body.

During Mark's first session, I evaluated him closely and found many, many problems. I tried not to overwhelm the family. I explained to Mark that therapy was going to be painful and tough, and he would need to understand it was the only way to reach the goals of being able to move in bed, sit upright, stand, and walk by himself. We started working three times a week; I blocked two full hours for him, even though I was busy in a management position within the PT department. I enjoyed working with Mark; he was always on time and ready to work hard at every session.

He was serious the first two weeks because I made him work very hard; however, he told me, "Keep doing the stretches, don't pay attention to my faces of pain." I stretched his hamstrings, fingers, wrists, elbows, shoulders, knees, ankles, and more. I was almost exhausted after every session, but it was a great feeling to see positive changes in his flexibility. The first time I put him on his stomach was like attempting to bend a piece of plywood. He was later able to tolerate more and more of his treatments. I could then start working with different groups of muscles.

Meanwhile, the family did incredibly well in following my instructions for working with Mark themselves.

Eventually, he sat normally in a wheelchair. On that day, my assistants and I felt good enough about his progress to set a date to stand him between the parallel bars.

I was in the front, one assistant was in the back and another on the side; it was a team effort, but we got him up. Mark was bent halfway over my chest, but he was up—after so many years. It was something to celebrate, and his family took pictures.

When he was able to roll over in bed, I wanted his best effort to help get him on his hands and knees, which is very painful for somebody with Mark's problems. Some days he behaved like a ten-year-old kid and wanted to play.

His parents warned me about him acting like a child, so I followed their advice to be resolute with him.

I was called in again to talk to him. He followed my instructions when I became more serious and listened more intently.

When he began to walk with a walker—another big goal—I offered to play chess with him. Amazingly, he could remember how to play chess and for many months told me he wanted me as a chess opponent. So I decided the competition would be excellent motivation for Mark. We bet that if *he* won we were going to take a break from physical therapy on that day, but if *I* won he was going to walk with the walker and follow all the instructions without playing around.

Mark accepted the challenge, and I won the bet. He was able to walk with the walker several times. I told him that, while I won the bet, he was the bigger winner because he could now walk with the walker—without assistance.

Several months later, Mark was able to walk using a quad cane with good, strong balance and was able to function independently in most of his daily activities. Shortly after he mastered the quad cane, he was ready to be discharged. His parents told me they were leaving with their "new" son to live on a small farm in North Carolina to enjoy the company of their son and explore their new life.

I hugged each one of them. Mark's mother gave me a big, warm hug. Knowing everything she had gone through to bring Mark back was very emotional for me; I felt tears rolling down my face. I knew this was going to be last time I would see them. Before they left, I remember talking to Mark, who was as happy as a kid in a candy store. He was excited about spending his new life on a farm with his parents.

It makes me happy to remember Mark's case, because when you have a busy practice you don't always realize the wonderful relationships life provides you.

CHAPTER FOUR

The Harley Guy

On a beautiful sunny day, Scott rode his motorcycle with his girlfriend on their way to Tampa. The I-4 drive was perfect—not too busy—but the problem was, he told me later, he'd had a few beers. He stopped near Orlando to see his buddies and decided to drink some beers with them. It was summer in Florida, and he believed drinking beer would be a good way to relax.

He had recently traded in his old bike for a new one, and he wanted to test it on the highway, which was a big mistake. Due to the speed and his unsteadiness with the new bike, Scott lost control. His girlfriend was lucky; she sustained only minor scratches and was able to get off the motorcycle and roll off the side of the lane.

Scott endured the worse part. He was still on the bike until it came to a complete stop after it slid for almost 500 feet. He felt his right lower leg against the pavement, caught underneath the motorcycle's burning-hot engine.

Aside from receiving multiple fractures, the severe burn almost destroyed his lower leg. His pain was excruciating, but the emergency crew was shocked to learn he was more concerned about the condition of his bike than his leg.

He was sent to a hospital in Tampa, which was closer, and upon admission had surgery due to the many fractures in his leg, arms, and ankles. He ended up losing his leg, which was the only option the surgeon had to save Scott's life. Amputations are very hard for everybody, but Scott had an amputation below the knee, which is one of the most functional amputations.

When he left the hospital, Scott came back home to south Florida to start his rehabilitation. That's when I saw him. He started on a Monday, which is one of the busiest days in all rehabilitation centers. He was not a nice person when I first met him.

Sometimes a person leaves their house without a care in the world, then suddenly one mistake makes a tremendous change in their life, which is what happened to Scott. When something traumatic happens, a patient like Scott goes through many stages. The first is shock, then crying or sorrow, unfortunately, then comes anger and hating everybody. Scott was upset and questioned God over and over, which is the stage he was in when I encountered him. Lucky me. The best phase was supposed to come next: to calm down, accept the situation, and start living life in the best way possible.

We had a long way to go.

Scott had many tattoos, and he was upset that his best tattoo was gone because of the amputation. He couldn't seem to focus on what was important to his recovery. His stump was healing, but it was still an open wound. It was imperative to heal the wound; otherwise, fitting for a prosthetic leg would be delayed, which would extend his recovery time. The whirlpool was the best choice for treatment, but it was a very small area, difficult to move around in.

Scott told me several times, "I am leaving . . . I can't do this . . . This is not for me . . . I am sorry, I can't!"

I insisted on talking to him very calmly, however, and made myself very clear. I told him that I understood his frustration with the whirlpool being very tight, but it was very important to try. I told him we were going to do his therapy as a team, and if we couldn't do it, I would let him go.

It wasn't easy, but we finally got it right.

After the treatment, Scott smiled a little. I asked him what he thought about it, and he told me even though it was a pain to get in and out of the whirlpool, he enjoyed it and relaxed once he was in.

His wound became clean, which was the best part, and we continued doing whirlpool therapy for several weeks until it closed. It was a great feeling of accomplishment for both of us. I cheered him up regularly and worked to make him understand the steps ahead.

In the meantime, Scott's friends from the local Harley Davidson group held all kinds of events to support him. I was invited and saw many good people who wanted to help Scott financially, since he couldn't work during his recovery. He was an independent contractor and even offered to build my house at that time.

The prosthetic leg was finally fitted, and he returned to me to start working with it. Scott was not too excited with the prosthetic at first, but I showed him that with effort and dedication, it would work. It was not so terrible for him, and he was surprised when he took the first few steps. He began very slowly using a walker, and within a week he could walk very fast. He got used to the prosthetic quickly. He had crossed a big hurdle: He was walking. We began to train for walking up and down stairs, curbs, then walking with only a cane. Later, he needed no assistive device at all. Scott seemed to reach his goals very easily.

He smiled and felt there was hope again, which I enjoyed witnessing. After only a few months, and because of his rapid progress, he was going to be discharged. He was happy and emotional at once, but he told me he was going to come back in one month.

It was a little strange for me because I didn't know what he was going to do when he came back. The month passed and one day my secretary told me Scott was on the phone for me. He sounded so excited, I could hear him laughing. I asked where he was, and he told me he was at a friend's bar! He said that in twenty minutes he was going to be at the clinic because he wanted to show me something.

I became a little nervous. I didn't know what to expect from his surprise, so I went back to work.

Scott showed up between patients. It was great to see him walk and move around without any problems. He said, "Come to the parking area and I'll show you my new toy."

We walked outside to the parking lot, and there it was: one of the most beautiful motorcycles I had ever seen. It was a shiny silver motorcycle with a side car. It was the only bike Scott could ride due to the amputated leg, but it meant the world to him. It represented completion of his therapy goal after many months of rehabilitation.

I didn't hear from him after that, but I knew his experience was a big lesson that changed him for the better.

So many traumatic situations can affect you. It reminds me that life is so short—a day-by-day fight to choose the right path—and when the night comes, it brings hope with the sunrise of a new day.

We see changes like Scott's very often when working in the physical therapy field. Life is altered for a patient after an accident or a disease.

CHAPTER FIVE

A New PT Treats the Wrong Patient

I once worked as the clinical director of physical therapy at a hospital in Florida. My role was management of the PT department as a whole, which included inpatient and outpatient services. It was very time consuming, but I enjoyed it. I had just completed my master's degree, and I wanted to put everything I had learned into practice to develop the best service possible. One of my duties was to interview potential employees. We were growing at a fast pace and needed to fill several positions as soon as possible.

One day, in came Nicole, a newly graduated PT from a prestigious college up north. She looked so young but had quite a personality. She had very limited experience in the inpatient setting; she said she had only a brief clinical rotation in a very small hospital. We needed help quickly, so I decided to hire her. But first I asked the senior staff to assist Nicole to make her transition and training go smoothly. I had to be sure the situation was comfortable for her and that the older staff members conducted themselves properly.

The senior staff was hard on new employees, especially the new young faces coming in with fresh knowledge. Many had just received a master's degree; the "old school" requirement was only a bachelor's of science. The senior staff helped her understand the hospital hierarchy. She was told she should follow their instructions. Once they saw Nicole could perform her job without supervision only a couple of weeks after her first day, they decided to let her do the rounds by herself on the cardiac floor.

With her new assignment, Nicole felt empowered. She said she knew she could perform professional work without the help of the senior staff. She felt she could finally put them in their places and demonstrate she was ready to work.

Her role was to work with patients assigned to her, which consisted mostly of basic therapy: therapeutic exercises in bed, showing the patients how to transfer in the safest possible way, and typical gait training. Once the patient masters gait training, they can move on to a rehab center or go directly home. It's why you see some patients walk the halls around the nursing station, over and over; their goal is to get out of the hospital as quickly as possible.

Nicole went to see her first patient on the cardiac floor and introduced herself. She did an assessment and began to treat her without any problems. The patient was cooperative but very weak.

While Nicole was in the room, she heard a commotion coming from outside of the room. It is quite common to hear equipment noises and voices from the speakers, so she didn't pay much attention. Besides, she knew she couldn't leave the room while working with a patient.

After a few minutes, the noise and commotion stopped; Nicole was pleased it was finally more quiet. She finished with her first patient and went to the nursing station, but nobody was there. That was unusual, and she was confused because she wasn't sure what had happened.

Nicole had work to do, so she prepared for her next patient, Mr. Jones. She found his medical chart on the counter and thought, *Great!* She reviewed the chart and read the last note written earlier, which told that Mr. Jones was very sick. So she simply followed her protocol and thought about range-of-motion exercises or anything similar that Mr. Jones might be able to tolerate.

She walked into the room to find the patient was unresponsive and a little colder than a regular patient. She introduced herself to Mr. Jones. "Good morning, Mr. Jones. I am your physical therapist, and I am going to move your legs and arms." She explained what she was going to do, describing to Mr. Jones the entire physiological and mechanical component of each exercise. It was really a monologue; Mr. Jones didn't speak or even open his eyes.

Nicole performed the therapeutic exercises for around twenty minutes and decided Mr. Jones had received enough range-of-motion exercises. She was exhausted; he hadn't cooperated at all. She felt good about the job she performed and left the room. At the nurse's station to return the chart, she saw quite a few people present. She thought to herself how weird it was not seeing anybody twenty to thirty minutes ago.

The head nurse was filling out a report and saw Nicole coming out of Mr. Jones' room and asked, "Who are you?"

Nicole, feeling good, replied, "Hi, I am the new physical therapist."

The room fell silent, and everyone stared at Nicole. The head nurse was at a loss for words but finally asked her, "Are you aware that Mr. Jones is dead? He died just a short time ago; the 'Code Blue' was called, but they were unable to resuscitate him."

In that moment, Nicole put all of the pieces together. First, the noises and voices coming from the speakers, which called the Code Blue Team. Second, no nurses in the nurse's station, and third—and the worst one—she had just treated a dead person! She almost fainted; it was entirely too much for her.

The nurses came to her defense, but she was already the subject of discussion among her peers in every single floor of the hospital.

Even writing this story is still somewhat funny and incredible. I feel sorry for her having to endure that awful experience. She was with us for two more months but left the hospital because she wanted to move away from a bad start.

When I train young therapists, I mention Nicole's story to them. Some don't believe me, others think it is possible if they don't pay attention. But the lesson is to communicate with the hospital staff before you do anything to a patient. I always did that, and I can't recall ever treating a dead person during my career.

CHAPTER SIX

Fire Ants!

I was working in a hospital on the Treasure Coast of Florida when we received a very unique and weighted piece of equipment for our PT department, the famous Hydrosound. It had a fancy name for what was actually a big tub; but, instead of a typical noisy whirlpool, the Hydrosound worked with bubbles that came from the ultrasound heads in the wall of its enormous tub. The staff was excited because it was so quiet, so much so that, when it first arrived, everyone thought it was broken. We were eager to put the new machine to real use.

It was dark when Mr. Sullivan went to check on something in his backyard: He wanted to see if he forgot to pick up all of his newspaper earlier that day. Parts of the newspaper were spread out over his table, but the wind had pushed the rest of the pages across the backyard.

Mr. Sullivan lived alone and was ninety-two years old. He maintained a very healthy lifestyle and tried to stay in shape as much as he could. Most of his family lived up north (like many of the families in south

Florida), and he didn't have many friends. But neighbors waved to him in the mornings when he walked around the neighborhood. It was summer, so his grass was long, despite the fact that the lawn service had already come earlier that week. With the rain and hot weather in Florida, the grass grows at a furiously fast pace. We also deal with large numbers of ants, especially fire ants, which are small red ants that can give you a lot of pain with their poisonous bites and stings if you don't pay attention to their mounds when you walk on the grass.

Around 7:30, it was still light enough outside to pick up his newspaper, so he rushed a little bit, he later told me, to get back to his favorite couch to watch a comedy and return to bed. He was so focused on getting the newspaper, he tripped over the long grass and took a horrible fall. He felt severe pain, probably from a twisted ankle. He said he knew he was falling down over the grass, so he thought the best way to land was to fall into it and get up fast. It was getting dark quickly.

Instead, his fall was hard and over something that he didn't expect. It wasn't just grass, it was something really bulky. Mr. Sullivan immediately realized it was a fire ant bed. He felt bites and stings on his foot, which was already painful from the twist and sprain of his ankle. Then the ants began to spread up to his knee, hip, genital area, abdomen, back, and eventually all over his body.

The pain was so terrible, and the ants were relentless. He was bitten over and over. It was by far the worst pain that somebody could experience. Mr. Sullivan was afraid for his life. He knew that his heart could stop and nobody would hear his cries for help. There was nothing else to do. He screamed in pain, but nobody could hear him, even though the houses in his neighborhood were only fifty feet apart. Because all the neighbors' AC units were on and their homes' windows and doors were closed, it was impossible for anyone to hear what was going on outside.

Mr. Sullivan estimated he had been lying there for twenty to thirty minutes, and the fire ants were still biting and stinging him, but less frequently. When the fire ants came to attack yet again, he tried to accommodate his injured back, which was also causing him pain.

Another thirty minutes passed before the ants calmed down. It was already dark, and Mr. Sullivan didn't know what to do. He felt his pulse racing and was beginning to have a panic attack. He prayed to God to help him since he was unable to do anything else. He knew if he could resist all his pain and fear until first light, one of his neighbors would find him when they came out to get their newspaper. He thought they would notice his newspaper, still in the driveway, which would be very unusual. He knew that would cause them to check on him. His problem was that he was in his *backyard*.

He couldn't resist anymore; he was in so much pain that for the next few hours he prayed to die. He was suffering from shock, and having too much poison in his body was causing intense pain.

The hours slowly passed by. He was losing the battle; he fainted and regained consciousness, over and over. Every time he opened his eyes, he thought it was already morning, but in reality it was only 1:00 AM, then 1:30 AM, and so on. By 6:00 he was unable to keep his eyes open, and he felt he was going to die. The ants were still biting and stinging him, but he was so weak that he couldn't feel his legs or his body anymore.

He was doing his best to save his last drops of energy just to stay awake. At 6:30, one of his neighbors, who always got up at that time to pick up his newspaper, noticed something was unusual: Mr. Sullivan's newspaper was still in the driveway. The neighbor could not remember ever having seen that before. He had always said to himself, *Mr. Sullivan always beats me by picking up his newspaper first.*

The good neighbor was worried; after all, Mr. Sullivan was in his nineties. He knocked on the front door and rang the doorbell, but nothing happened. He knocked on the door, again with no response. Then he panicked, wondering, *What if something bad has happened?* He walked to the back of the house to see if a window or one of the doors were open. *All closed.*

As he walked toward the backyard he saw something—or somebody—lying on the grass. He moved closer and saw Mr. Sullivan unconscious with hundreds of fire ants crawling over his body. The neighbor immediately called 911.

Emergency medical services personnel responded extremely fast and carefully placed Mr. Sullivan on the stretcher. They were stunned to see that he was still showed vital signs. He was still alive!

Once at the hospital, the emergency room team rushed to counteract the ant poison and provide him comfort. The doctors couldn't believe he was alive or that his heart could survive so many hours of torture. He had presented with red marks and swelling all over his body; the fire ants had no mercy on him.

Mr. Sullivan received many IV treatments and antibiotics during his hospital stay. Part of his treatment was the debridement of damaged skin tissue from his body.

It was finally everyone's chance to see the Hydrosound in action. The Hydrosound water, mixed with the prescribed medicine, performed well and allowed us to treat all those bites and injuries without any discomfort to Mr. Sullivan. The power of ultrasound in water gently cleaned his body. It shocked us to see the amount of his skin and mucus floating in the water

In a week he demonstrated an amazing recovery. By the second week he was ready to transfer to a rehab facility. We were all happy to see him stronger and able to move better before he left us.

He constantly thought that he was not going to make it, but he survived, and it looked as if he was lucky the Hydrosound water treatment was available—just for him.

After that awful experience, I always advise my patients to be extremely careful when they go out in the dark. This is one story you don't want to experience first hand.

CHAPTER SEVEN

A 101-Year-Old Man
Gets a Traffic Ticket

Years ago, I co-owned a physical therapy office with a colleague. We offered free transportation to our patients who
were unable to drive their car to our office or didn't have
anyone to bring them. A community bus came by, but not frequently,
and it was difficult for patients to adjust to its schedule. We sent our
driver to pick up patients and take them back to their houses very
quickly and safely. The patients always enjoyed that.

Our transportation service was a good way to help patients
and also attract business. And it's how we came to care for Alfred,
a gentleman of 101 years of age. He had suffered a fall and was
recovering from a shoulder fracture. He couldn't drive, not only
because of the fracture, but because of his advanced age. He was
a very funny man. During his first session he made us laugh with
his humor and stories. The following story was told by him and his
family to us.

Six months earlier, when he was 100 years old, Alfred chose to keep his 1980's model Ford Lincoln, twenty years old at the time. It was in good condition because it was a one-owner car he drove only from his house to church or the supermarket—or anywhere that wasn't one-and-a-half miles too far from his home.

The family worried about his driving, but at the same time they felt a bit more comfortable knowing that he had driven close to home for years. One morning he took his car and drove from his house to the supermarket. He had to take the hectic route and drove on U.S. Highway 1 for approximately one mile.

As he parked his car in the parking lot of the store, he hit another car at a very slow speed. But the other car, a small new Japanese model, was in bad shape. Nothing happened to Alfred or the other driver, but the police were called and arrived at the scene very quickly.

A crowd began to form outside of the supermarket to see what was going on. Several police cars drove in. Alfred thought they were crazy to have so many police officers show up, but at the same time he thought they could just be hungry and for breakfast wanted to get some donuts or something like that from the store.

About a half hour later, a policeman approached Alfred and said, "Sir, I want to ask you a few questions."

"Yes, what do you need to know?" Alfred replied, very sure of himself.

The policeman, with an embarrassed and amused look on his face, asked Alfred, "How old are you?"

Alfred responded with an upset tone, "One hundred years old. What is wrong with that?"

The policeman said, "Well, you cannot drive a vehicle at that age, sir. There is no way the state will allow you to do that, so we are going to have to confiscate your driver's license. We are calling your son to come and get you."

Alfred was furious; they had taken his driver's license away.

In Florida, like other communities, a driver's license is a person's independence. While a police officer, a judge, physician or even a family member can take that away from you, it can hurt your pride, your independence, and your freedom. It can be very tough for some patients to come to terms with. I have seen patients who realize they are too old to drive and give their license away of their own choice. But for others, like Alfred, there was no way anyone was going to stop him from driving his car.

His son, who knew Alfred well, had also taken his car away from him because he knew his father was going to attempt to continue driving—with or without a license.

Alfred was very disappointed when his car was taken, but having no license and no car, he thought, *Well, I still can get around; I have my golf cart.*

One morning, instead of waiting for his family to take him to the supermarket, he just took off in his golf cart and drove all the way to the entrance of U.S. Highway 1.

In that area of the highway, the speed limit is forty-five to fifty-five miles per hour: one section is fifty-five, then, close to the supermarket, forty-five. A golf cart moves at a very slow speed and is quite a fragile vehicle. It is against the law to take a golf cart on the road where cars are.

After they almost hit him, many drivers furiously honked their horns and flashed their lights to get his attention. It was a spectacle. Everybody shouted at him, "Get off the road!"

Alfred didn't care; he just continued in the right lane of U.S. Highway 1 on his way to the store.

The trip seemed to take forever, he recalled. But he lucked out when the police stopped him. Alfred saw the car, but he acted as if he didn't see it and continued to drive without stopping.

Another police car and then another joined the first police car. Soon, five police cars followed Alfred's golf cart. At one point, the police used a loudspeaker to say, "Sir, stop at once!"

Alfred continued driving.

After fifteen minutes there was another commotion in the parking lot of the supermarket. He had just parked the golf cart when all the police who were not too happy with him came to arrest him.

Alfred continued to pretend to be oblivious to the situation. "Excuse me, officer, but what happened?" Alfred innocently asked.

The cops were irritated but laughed.

Alfred's son was called again, but this time the police warned him, "If this happens again, we will take your father to jail."

His son took away Alfred's golf cart, and he was upset that he lost all means of transportation.

Alfred did great with his therapy; his shoulder returned to full function within a few weeks. He also was able to run the treadmill like my younger patients. I enjoyed every session with him. He was really funny, not because he wanted you laugh about those things, but because he was so serious when he told his stories.

The driving scenario happens a lot, of course, not always with the same intensity as Alfred's, but most of our elderly population are just "waiting for that damn day" when they lose their driver's license because of old age.

CHAPTER EIGHT

Falls

U nfortunately, falls are very frequent in the senior population. Government, insurance companies, and other entities have worked for years to decrease the percentage of falls. Here, in Florida, it is extremely common because of our large retirement community.

Throughout the years, I have heard the most incredible stories relating to falls. I would like to share three, hoping the experiences of others can help the reader understand why we as physical therapists believe so strongly about safety and precautions as part of our plan of care with every single patient.

We need to be more proactive; instead, we are *reactive* after the problem is already present. Our role as physical therapists is to instruct, in a very conservative way, for patients to avoid falls. If taught properly, patients will know what to do.

The High Heels

Years ago I saw a very nice lady, Miranda, who had just undergone surgery to fix a broken femur, the thigh bone. Surgery consisted of affixing a plate and pins, and as a result, she was unable to bear weight on the leg for eight weeks. She was sent to an in-patient rehabilitation center to recover. She came home after two long months of misery and a tough time recovering because of her awful fall. That is when I met her.

Miranda lived alone in a second-floor condominium. She was happy she had bought the apartment, which was in a quiet community that featured a nice pool and many gardens. She was only fifty-six years old and was by far the youngest in the community. Her neighbors frequently asked her for help, and she willingly helped them. She was happy to take her elderly friends to doctors' appointments or shopping. It gave her an opportunity to dress up and wear her high heels, which she loved. She had worn them for years.

It was summer in Florida, which is hurricane season. The previous year's storm caused her whole condominium to have a power outage for almost a week, which made it impossible to cook, wash, dry, or anything else that required electricity. Miranda refused to go through another hurricane season unprepared; this year she was prepared and watchful of the weather reports so she could anticipate any problems. Therefore, it was easy for her when she heard on her car's radio about a new storm coming.

This time, she vowed, *the storm is not going to surprise me.*

She washed her clothes right away instead of waiting until the storm approached the area. She thought it was a brilliant idea, so she grabbed all of her dirty clothes and began her first load. When the first load was finished, Miranda started to wash her second load. After the second load was going, she passed a mirror, paused, and thought about even washing the clothes that she was wearing. Since there wasn't anyone around, she did it.

She wore only her high heels, which were over five inches high. She had never changed her shoes since she came from shopping. Suddenly, she remembered she needed to get clothes from the other room. She moved very quickly and almost ran from room to room to find other clothes to throw in with her next load. While searching for clothes, she discovered a problem. A bit of water was on the tile from the wet laundry.

It was a terrible combination, high heels and running. Miranda said she felt as if she were suddenly flying through the air like a ballerina when she slipped in the water. One leg went forward and the other went backward. In that second she knew that something bad was going to happen. She fell in a perfect split; however, her right hip made an awful sound, and she blacked out.

Thirty minutes passed. Miranda was naked, wearing only her high heels. Her right leg was crooked, and she was in excruciating pain. She was close by her phone but couldn't move to reach it because the pain was too severe. She desperately needed to reach the phone to call for help. She pressed her courage, grabbed her leg with both hands, and tried to position it correctly. Unfortunately, she fainted again due to the severity of the pain.

After fifteen minutes she woke up again, but this time she decided to move as close as she could to the phone. The only problem was that her phone was at the top of the kitchen counter. Miranda thought if she could pull the cord first, she would be able to pull the phone to her. She attempted to reach the phone at least five times—between the pain and the fainting—until finally she was able to reach it.

The first person Miranda called was *not* 911 but her girlfriend next door, who she asked to come and help her dress before the emergency crew arrived. I still have no idea how her friend was able to get her dressed due to her twisted leg and the severity of her pain, but she did it.

Miranda proved that style was important!

The lesson to be learned is to be extremely careful when you wear unstable shoes because they can cause severe injuries as you get older.

The Lady Without a Real Family

Dorothy was a happy and independent lady who lived alone in her house. She was a quiet woman but happy to be comfortable in her retirement years. She had seven children, six of whom lived five to twenty minutes away from her house, and one son who lived out of state.

Ironically, she was left alone. She didn't have any pets or a caregiver, and none of her nearby kids visited her—but she regularly called them. They never tried to stay in contact with her, so Dorothy ended up not calling them after time. She knew if they needed something they would call her for assistance, so she carried on with her life.

Her son was in Atlanta, Georgia and was the only one who stayed in touch with her. Once every two weeks he talked to Dorothy on the phone. She didn't go out too much, mainly to go to the supermarket. Her neighbors knew about her, but they knew very little about her family situation.

One afternoon, Dorothy felt some discomfort in her head and chest. She thought that it was a simple headache so didn't give it a second thought. She continued with her activities of the day. She thought the pain would improve after a night's rest.

The next morning, when she needed to go to the bathroom, she got up and carefully took a few steps. *The pain is not so bad*, she thought to herself. Unfortunately, she fainted and fell down the stairs, hitting both her head and her hip on the tile floor.

Dorothy broke her leg, but the reason for her fall was a stroke.

She lay on the floor, waiting for someone to come help. She didn't have a personal alarm system and could not reach the phone. Hers was a "Floridian floor," a very strong floor that is tougher and cooler than modern tile. Older Florida houses used Floridian floors as a way to compensate for having no air conditioning.

She was on the floor for an entire day and recalled praying and waiting for somebody to come to her rescue. But hours passed, and nobody came. She was thirsty, extremely weak, unable to move her left side, and felt a horrific pain in her right hip.

The next day, her whole body was numb, and she knew it was only a matter of time before her body would fail. She passed out and was unconscious for the next couple of days.

Her son from Georgia called several times, with no answer. He immediately worried because he never before had any problems reaching her. He tried calling again later, thinking she could possibly be running errands. He tried in the evening, and still no answer. He was certain something had happened to his mother, so he called the local police and one of his brothers in the area. The local brother phoned her mother's neighbor, who noticed Dorothy's newspapers and mail were accumulating, which she had never seen happen.

The neighbor knocked on the door, but there was no answer. The police came and opened the main door. No lights were on. When they turned on the light they could see a body on the floor. The poor woman had been lying there for five long days!

The police called for an ambulance. The paramedics thought she was dead, but to their surprise she still had a pulse—weak, but it was something for her to grip onto for dear life. Once hospitalized, she showed signs of recovery. It was like a miracle.

The stroke had beaten Dorothy badly, and she had been unconscious for many days and without food and water. The damage was permanent: right-sided numbness and paralysis. She underwent hip surgery due to the severity of the fracture. She made it through the entire recovery process and finally went home.

While Eorothy's hip was repaired, the stroke had taken its toll. She was able to perform transfers and gait training—a miracle due to the damage from her stroke. She made it and moved back home, fighting against all odds. She was dehydrated, suffered with a fixed hip, and lived alone after having had a stroke.

The state intervened in Dorothy's tragic case and agreed to make a caregiver available for her. Her local children, however, never showed up. The only one of her children to visit was her son from Georgia. He had always come to visit her when he could.

Dorothy's was a sad story, but it showed me how strong a person's will to survive can be. She was definitely able to show me her inner strength every singe day I had the opportunity to be her therapist.

A Fall in the Shower

I've spent many years listening to stories about falling in the shower or in the kitchen, which are the two main areas it normally happens, because of tile or wet floors. But the story of a fall that moved me the most was Alice's story.

Alice lived alone in her house and was a very strong and independent woman. She was very active in the community and maintained a busy schedule filled with activities, such as shopping, church, and a bridge group. On Saturdays, Alice went to the beauty parlor. She was a customer in the same parlor for many years and knew the entire staff. Her appointment was always on the same day and time of the week, and she never missed a day, which may have saved her life.

One Friday early afternoon, she returned home from shopping and decided to take a shower. It was summer, and she'd spent a long, hot morning out. *A nice shower will cool me down*, Alice reasoned. So she prepared everything and got into the shower.

She didn't have a walk-in-shower, but she got in without any difficulty. Alice was enjoying the water when she dropped her bar soap, leaned forward to pick it up, and slipped so badly she hit her head on the wall. She fell backward, twisting her left leg. Just before she passed out she heard a very strange sound; something broke in her hip.

She woke up after a few seconds and didn't know what to do. She experienced severe pain in her hip. The water was still running in the shower and spraying directly on her. Alice couldn't move and had forgotten to take the precaution of always having easy access to a phone, something she'd always heard about from family members and friends. Her phones were in her bedroom and living room, very far from where she was. After fifteen or twenty minutes, the water was getting colder; she knew that she had to act quickly.

She was able to move her other leg, but the pain was so severe she was afraid to move. The water got colder and colder. She knew if she stayed where she was she could get hypothermia, which she knew was very dangerous. Alice thought the situation was ironic since it was quite hot outside. After a few attempts, Alice was able to stop the water using her good foot. It was a big accomplishment, and she was excited she could do it. But she couldn't move any farther than she already had, and her pain had intensified.

She thought, *Somebody will call, maybe my son or a friend.* Then she thought, *Why would they call me?* She had just spoken with her son earlier and saw her friends yesterday. She began to feel desperate.

It was already night, and she was very cold, wet, and naked in the bathtub—with a broken hip. She needed to do something to get her body warm or to cover up with something. Then Alice thought, *The shower curtains! They are plastic and vinyl but could help.* She pulled them down and covered herself with them. Her back was also injured, and the pain of it had become excruciating. She could no longer move.

Alice was "at God's mercy," as she described it to me. The hours passed very slowly. She didn't know exactly what time it was; she had no clock or a watch nearby. She prayed for someone to come by, but nobody came. She tried to sleep. No lights were on; the only source of light was very faint and from the moon shining through a small window.

Many thoughts came to her mind. She was so upset with herself. She'd heard all the stories and advice from her loved ones, but she never paid any attention. Now, Alice was paying for that and learning her lesson the hardest of ways. She decided upon the steps she needed to take to survive. One was to get some sleep. She tried to close her eyes to sleep but shivered with cold. The shower curtain was not helping her well enough, and the air conditioning unit kicked on quite often.

When she had come back that day from shopping, she had

adjusted the thermostat down to seventy-three degrees. (She told me she normally put it back close to eighty at night so she wouldn't get cold). It was a horrible experience for her, shivering and trying to not move due to excruciating pain.

The first signs of morning finally came. More light shone in her window, and Alice could see her situation more clearly. She didn't have any clue about the day or time; she assumed it was Saturday. The only thing she had scheduled was the beauty parlor at 10:00.

When she didn't show up for her appointment and never called, the hairdresser, who knew her for years, took notice. She instinctively knew something was wrong, so she picked up the phone and called Alice. Alice's phone rang and rang with no answer. The hairdresser became even more concerned and called Alice's son, who lived in the area. She asked him about his mother, and he said, "She *has* to be at home." The hairdresser insisted he check on her because, as she told the son, "Something is definitely not right." He went to his mother's house right away and opened the door with the extra key he had.

She finally felt relief when she heard him open the front door. *I'm going to make it.*

Her son found her in the shower, covered by the curtains and shivering. He called 911 and gave her towels and a blanket to warm up and cover up before the emergency crew came.

Alice learned her lesson. She had an alarm system installed and from then on carried a phone with her everywhere she went.

PTs constantly encounter cases like Alice's. It is important to be independent, but that independence needs to be combined with common sense and safety. Life can turn so quickly; one mistake can affect the rest of one's life. I have even known a patient who broke her neck in a fall after trying to step on a small stool while cleaning her home's curtains before Christmas. You would think that it was a very common and simple thing to do, to step on a stool, but one misstep can bring such severe consequences, such as paralysis.

It is important to continue to discuss the subject of home safety to promote a healthy and safe life for every individual.

CHAPTER NINE

Hurricane Stories

We live in Florida, and aside from the beaches, sun, tropical fruits, big cities, and tourism, we have something that causes us to be on guard every year from June to the end of November: hurricane season. Through my career, I have been through five hurricanes in this area. And some of my patients have had the most incredible stories to tell, including the following three.

The Hearing Aid

Mr. Smith was a very friendly old man who lived with his wife in a nice inland location, which means the beach was about six miles from their house. Mr. Smith was improving from knee surgery and was able to move around very well with walker in his house. He was ready to start his gait training with a regular cane.

News channels bombarded us about a big hurricane that had formed in the Atlantic Ocean, and every single one of us were paying attention—too much, maybe. But it was the first real threat of a hurricane coming toward the area, and it seemed our town was going to be ground zero.

Mr. Smith had a daughter who lived in the area and who was very involved with his care. She thought about how her poor parents would fare, alone in the storm. *Nobody can travel later*, she thought, *because the National Guard will establish a curfew for the whole area.* So, she went to her parents' house to stay with them while the storm passed.

Mr. Smith decided not to put any shutters on his windows. He always said that every single year they scare you about storms, but nothing ever happens. *Besides*, he reasoned, *this year I'm recovering from knee surgery.* It was the perfect excuse.

His wife agreed, but she wasn't entirely convinced.

Night came, and the three had an early dinner as the wind and rain started to increase.

After dinner, Mr. Smith became tired and went to bed. Following his routine, Mr. Smith got in bed and removed his hearing aids. He placed his head on the pillow and fell asleep very quickly.

His wife and daughter began to move from the living room to another area of the house in preparation for the long, stormy night ahead. An hour later, the wind whipped the rain very strongly. The electricity went out; darkness enveloped everything. Mother and daughter carried flashlights, but the noise of the wind and rain was so deafening they could barely hear each other.

They were scared and prayed for safety. They checked on Mr. Smith to see if he was scared like they were. They could barely believe he was sleeping like a baby! The windows sounded like they were ready to break with each gust of wind. The women were so concerned they decided to stay close to Mr. Smith's room in case they needed to rescue him from a broken window. He just slept peacefully on his bed, despite all the noise.

They chose to stay in Mr. Smith's closet and shared the very tight small place. They prayed and hoped the storm would move away. The wind increased with each gust, and they thought everything was going to blow to pieces. Mrs. Smith began to think her biggest mistake was letting her husband convince her not to put up the shutters this year.

The hours passed very slowly, and it was almost first light the next day when the storm showed signs of weakening. Both women were exhausted, not just physically but mentally. They opened the closet and thanked God nothing bad had happened to them.

Twenty minutes later, Mr. Smith woke up with a big smile on his face, and he did what normally did: He put in his hearing aids then asked his wife and daughter, "What happened to you two?"

They couldn't believe it. He couldn't hear anything last night without his hearing aids!

It took me three days after the storm to see Mr. Smith again, and I asked his wife how the experience had affected him.

"I can't believe he was able to sleep so well that night," she told me and went on to describe their ordeal and how he'd slept right through it.

Mr. Smith's natural state of being hard of hearing was definitely a blessing for him that night.

The Boat

Mr. Tomasewski lived in a beautiful house by the waterfront in a very nice neighborhood. He and his wife loved the location. He had a great boat at his own dock. Life was perfect in every way he could see it. The problem was the bad weather.

He, like every Floridian, knew a hurricane was predicted to come to the area. Mr. Tomasewski was optimistic and thought that, at the last minute, the storm would veer to a different direction.

He and his wife decided to visit a friend who lived about forty-five minutes from their house. As they left for their friend's house, they encountered very light traffic, but people were running from store to store to stock up on supplies to ride out the storm. The aftermath of a storm is almost worse than the storm itself because of power outages and closed businesses.

They were having a nice lunch with their friend and didn't want to pay attention to the news, but after their meal they heard from others that they should go back to their house as soon as possible because curfew would start in thirty minutes. The storm was definitely moving to this area.

They left in their car, and Mr. Tomasweski realized the only way he would beat the curfew was to speed. He told his wife to close her eyes if she wanted because he was going to drive fast. No cars were on the road, but from time to time they saw the National Guard. When Mr. Tomasewski told me his speed was one hundred miles per hour, my jaw dropped.

They made it home just before the wind and the rain started coming down very hard. Once inside the house, he thought about his boat. He could see it moving back and forth, side to side, and hitting his dock. He wanted to do something about it, but his wife insisted he should leave it alone and avoid doing anything foolish. After all, she reminded him, they'd made it safely home after driving one hundred miles per hour.

Mr. Tomasweski couldn't bear the idea of his boat being directly in the storm's path and being torn apart from being tied down too tightly as the water rose. He turned to his wife and said, "What about tying a long rope around my waist and holding the end of it so I can get safely to the boat and cut the support?"

His wife thought it was a crazy, stupid idea, but he convinced her. He took a long rope from the garage and did just what he described. The wind was so strong he could take only a few steps without falling. Willpower alone helped him reach the boat, but by then the boat was receiving the full impact of the water and the wind. He cut some rope but fell down. He was able to get up but was afraid and chose to leave the boat alone. It was too late; his back was already strained. He struggled painfully to get back to his house, which he could just barely see. Behind him, his boat was being taken down by the waves and strong wind! Mr. Tomasweski came to my physical therapy office five days after the hurricane with a diagnosis of lumbar strain. He didn't tell me much in the beginning, but I asked about the rope marks on his back. He confessed the craziness he'd gone through. The ironic part was that in a week he received a nice check from his boat insurance that paid for it without any further questions.

I told him, "You almost lost your life for nothing, because the boat insurance paid you right away."

Hopefully, his lesson was learned.

The Cat

Mr. McDougall lived alone at ninety-two years of age. He owned a nice mobile home, which is very common in our area. He lived in a well-known trailer park and enjoyed the tranquility. His only son lived in Arizona, and his only company was his faithful cat of ten years.

The cat was somewhat anti-social, maybe a little bit like Mr. McDougall, who suffered for many years with hip and low back pain. His doctor sent him home with orders for home health care, including PT, which was how I met him. He was in favor of therapy and was very cooperative during each session. He gained strength and the confidence to control his back pain. He progressed quickly and reported minimal pain.

Then along came the crazy week one hurricane moved dangerously close to our area.

Local authorities were overwhelmed with preparations before the storm arrived. It came time for mandatory evacuation of the entire trailer park; everybody had to leave, and they were instructed go to a relative's home, a shelter, or another area.

I advised Mr. McDougall to obey local authorities and leave early to avoid the chaos of leaving at the last minute. He had my cell phone number so we could be in touch after the hurricane if a connection were available.

I was evacuating with my family to the north when I received his call.

"Mr. McDougall, I thought you had already left the area," I said, alarmed that he was still at home.

He told me no, he hadn't because his cat could not go with him—and he wouldn't go anywhere without his cat.

It was too late to go in person to help him, so I called a friend who was a certified nurse assistant who also saw Mr. McDougall for his back. I explained the whole situation to her, and she assured me she would check on him.

When she arrived at Mr. McDougall's house, he was seated in his recliner, waiting for help. She realized his cat was in the bathroom and said there was no way to take it out because it was acting wild; it instinctively knew something was happening. She called animal control, but nobody answered, then she called 911 and explained that Mr. MacDougall needed to evacuate, he had everything in his car, but he wouldn't leave without his cat.

Emergency services sent out a lady with experience in that type of situation. She came to catch the cat and put him in the cage, walked into the bathroom, and closed the door. A series of crashes, meows, scratching, and other strange noises followed. She emerged empty handed.

"I need to get my gloves," she announced and went to her car. She returned wearing gloves that covered her hands and forearms all the way up to her elbows.

She walked inside the bathroom and closed the door again. It was possible to hear noises of the cat running from corner to corner, but this time with more intensity. The lady knew she would catch the cat and finally came out with the cat inside the cage. She looked as if she just came from a big fight.

Mr. McDougall happily left with his cat for the west coast of Florida. He told me that, on his way over, in the middle of nowhere, one of his tires went flat, so he just sat and waited for help. He was extremely lucky when a couple of young men stopped and replaced the tire.

He ended up staying several days in a hotel close to Tampa.

After the hurricane subsided, Mr. McDougall returned home with his cat. His trailer had very little damage, and he was very happy.

We continued with his therapy, but after a few weeks *another* hurricane had us in its sights. This time, Mr. McDougall didn't want to have the same experience and decided to go to a shelter. He left the cat behind in the trailer for a few days. He thought it would be okay and left plenty of food and water.

The hurricane passed, and he came home—to find a changed cat. The poor animal was in a corner of his bedroom, still shivering. He was very upset because his cat acted strangely . . . docile.

I said, "Who knows what the poor cat went through? The noises, the wind, and the lighting would be very scary for the cat, especially being alone."

He took very good care of his pet. After a week or so, it returned to its normal behavior.

What an awful year it was, and what a mess it left everywhere!

Stories of pets during storms are very common, and I have heard many others, but this one was very special. It highlighted the significance of one relationship between a person and an animal.

CHAPTER TEN

The Easter Weekend of Tragedy and Hope

The Miller family was happy to receive Mr. Miller's sister Anne and her husband for a visit on Easter weekend. The Millers were in their early thirties with two kids, a nine-year-old boy and a seven-year-old girl. They loved their Aunt Anne and were excited she was coming to spend a few days with them. It was going to be a great weekend to enjoy time together as a family and to have a break from a bitter weather affecting their home in the northeast.

They arrived on a Thursday, and the kids and family enjoyed the days with various activities. Mr. Miller was very excited to see his older sister and her husband, who were always very busy. Both had very demanding jobs and led very active social lives. They didn't have any kids, so the relationship they had with their niece and nephew was very special.

On Easter Sunday morning, they left for church early; they had a flight out booked for later that day. Mr. Miller took his van, and everybody piled in. Mr. and Mrs. Miller sat in the first row, Aunt Anne and her husband sat in the second row, and in the last row sat the two kids. It was 7:30, and church was just a few blocks away. They took a quiet, two-lane road. Nobody wore a seatbelt; they never thought anything would ever happen.

From the opposite direction came an old couple in their Cadillac. The speed limit was thirty-five miles per hour, and there were about 200 feet before the two vehicles would cross. Suddenly, the old man dropped something onto the floorboard, and his wife—the driver—leaned forward to pick it up. Without paying attention to the road, she turned her steering wheel, accidentally pressed the gas pedal, and the Cadillac ran head on into the Miller's van, crushing it in half.]

EMS was called by witnesses who were close by.

The old couple wore their seatbelts and sustained minor injuries, such as bumps, lacerations, and a sprained ankle—but nothing else.

Unfortunately, Mr. Miller flew through the windshield and hit the other car, and he had an open skull fracture. Although his wife was next to him in the vehicle, she didn't hit the other car, she hit the pavement and also had a brain injury. Aunt Anne didn't fly out of the van and neither did her husband, due to the seats in front of them. They had multiple fractures but no brain injuries. The kids also sustained injuries: one had a broken arm, the other a broken leg.

The young doctor in charge of the closest emergency room was happy the weekend had been calm. He hoped the day would end that way; however, he was completely wrong, it was going to be one of his worst days and busiest by far.

Everyone from the Miller wreck was taken to his ER, and the young doctor worked like never before. The two parents were in critical condition, but Mr. Miller was in the worst shape. He was in the same room with the rest of his family, lying one next to the other on different stretchers. Mr. Miller had brain matter protruding from his skull fracture. The doctor was shocked when Mr. Miller reached out and took his hand.

He opened his eyes, asking, "How are my kids?"

"They are okay, they are alive," the doctor reassured him.

Mr. Miller closed his eyes and passed away right then and there.

When I later talked to the doctor, he told me it had been a

miracle. There was no way, due to the injuries and brain damage, Mr. Miller could have opened his eyes and asked that question, but he did.

Miracles *do* happen.

Mrs. Miller was sent to another hospital after she was cleaned of debris by the young doctor's staff. After she was stabilized in the ER, she was sent to another hospital, four hours away by car. The doctors in both hospitals had been amazed at how her body fought to stay working, but she couldn't resist and also died.

A few days later, with both parents dead, Aunt Anne took over caring for the family. She couldn't believe what was happening. She too had to go for surgery; both her arm and shoulder were fractured, and her ankle was broken in four places.

She prayed to recover quickly so she could help those poor kids, who now were orphans. Her husband suffered multiple fractures in his thigh bone, the femur. Doctors were ready to amputate, but one surgeon felt confident enough to attempt a salvage of the leg. Both surgeries went well, and Aunt Anne soon asked to be sent home with the kids.

I was busy as the clinical director of physical therapy in the same hospital, so I'd already heard about the tragedy. The hospital staff was still in shock. The tranquility of a small town and community had been altered after the awful accident.

I received a call from a home health agency representative, who asked if I would work with a family of three or four—survivors of the accident I'd heard so much about.

I accepted right away. I don't know why I did it without doubts, since I was already so busy with many other responsibilities, but I felt one of those vibes: I knew I had to go.

I arrived to see Anne, who opened the door and moved in a wheelchair. She couldn't put any weight on the injured foot and, on her opposite side, the arm and shoulder were also recovering from surgery. She also had multiple rib fractures and other, more minor issues.

The pain of it all didn't stop Anne from doing her job and attending to her new responsibilities as a parent. She did amazingly well with therapy; I couldn't believe how well. I could see the pain in her face as she worked to recover, but she continued doing each activity until she finished it.

She told me many times, "I have to do this. They [the kids] have nobody except me and my husband." She worried when her husband developed an infection after the surgery and his blood pressure became unstable. In fact, he was still in the ICU. The kids each had their fractures casted and were able to move around. I could see they were still digesting the trauma of losing both parents.

Anne had a very difficult task before her. In the middle of therapy, after a few sessions, she opened up more and began to talk about her fears and the pressure, as well as her own sorrow, and her hope for the kids. She frequently cried, as you can imagine, and she questioned God, *Why?*

She didn't have kids of her own, but now she had two: her niece and nephew. She felt guilty in some way. But, she was amazing; she recovered from her weaknesses and became a strong woman ready to fight for her husband and those children.

Finally, her husband was able to come home. He was still in shock from the accident, the surgeries and an extended stay in the hospital, but he was happy to be back with his wife. To stabilize the fractures, the doctor attached a long plate that covered almost the whole thigh bone.

While Anne and the kids recovered very quickly from their fractures, her husband took longer. After home care, he came to the outpatient clinic to work with me. He was a model patient who became so strong that, from starting in a wheelchair, he was eventually able to walk with a cane outside of the house. He didn't need it inside.

Though years have passed, I still remember that family. I know the love of the aunt and uncle created hope from a tragedy. Sometimes I think such situations are an example to the rest of us. I always wear a seatbelt, even if I go somewhere only a block away. The other very important thing to remember is you never know when your life can change. Like the old saying: "Tomorrow is a mystery, but today is a gift!"

CHAPTER ELEVEN

New PT in Trouble!

I was in my last rotation for my professional practice. My class was working in a hospital under the teaching and supervision of a physiatrist, an MD who specialized in rehabilitation. He was quite strict and made us study extra hard to prepare for meetings he held with us just prior to assignment of the patients.

He was very short in stature and, to compensate, wanted us to fear him. He often made our lives miserable, especially the last three months before our graduation. I never studied much those days, but I didn't want to fail, and he pushed me to succeed.

I did quite well, so after a while he turned his attention to my classmates. The PT department featured a big room divided with curtains to create separate cubicles in which to treat the patients. We saw all kinds of patients with different diagnoses but mostly back pain, perhaps related to the local mining industry. It was very common to use heat as the first choice to treat someone who came in with back pain, and at that time we employed the use of moist heat pads or the infrared light.

Sophia was a bright student in our group but was forgetful at times. We always encouraged her to focus and be sharp, particularly during our last clinical last rotation.

One afternoon, she began treating a patient who came in with severe lumbar pain. He was exhausted and hadn't been able to sleep for several days. Finally, he came to receive therapy for the first time.

Sophia evaluated him and decided her plan of care was to concentrate on the pain as soon as possible for the poor man. She applied various modalities to control pain, which provided him some relief. She placed him on his stomach over the table and applied the infrared light.

He was in pain at the beginning of his treatment, but he reported the benefits quickly—stating he felt much better—then fell asleep after five minutes. Sophia didn't want to interrupt him and completed her paperwork. She stepped out of the cubicle and attended to another patient.

She finished with the other patient at 5:00 PM, quitting time. Everybody got ready to leave, and because we had a big exam the next day, Sophia was the first to go. She went to the library to pick up a book related to the next day's exam. Then everybody left, and the treatment area became quiet. The doctor in charge of us was still completing paperwork. Normally, he left between 5:30 and 6:00 PM.

Sophia was so tired after studying and work that as soon as she got home she fell asleep within a few minutes. Around midnight she woke up sweating and almost screaming. It was a nightmare. She thought there was no way this could happen to her: She forgot about her new patient in that cubicle, and he was under the infared light!

My God! The patient may already be burned! she thought.

She knew she would be in a lot of trouble—not only her but the doctor and the dean, as well. She called the hospital, but nobody answered. She got up and went to the hospital, but the security guard told her the whole area was closed and she should come back the next day.

She didn't sleep the whole night. She arrived early the next morning and went to check if her patient was still there.

Thank God he isn't! she almost shouted out loud when she found the cubicle empty.

She talked to me about the incident; I was the president of the class, so she thought there might be something I could do to help her.

I told her there wasn't much I could do, but I advised her to be honest and explain exactly how it happened so the situation wouldn't be worse for her.

She was extremely nervous.

The famous doctor came and before the meeting asked which PT student had left a patient in the treatment area.

Sophia did what I told her, jumped up right away, and said, "It was me."

The doctor asked her to step in his office. Wow! You could cut the tension with a knife. We heard the raised voice of the doctor as he yelled at her, again and again.

Sophia played her role well that day, she held her head down and just allowed the physiatrist to be very tough on her, because at the end he told her, "If this happens one more time, you are out of this profession!" He was tough, but she was okay with enduring the situation because she learned the patient had not been injured.

The physiatrist told her that, as he prepared to leave at 5:30, he saw a weird red light coming from one of the cubicles. He checked and found the patient sleeping in a prone position under the light, which the doctor turned off. Luckily, the patient was only red from all the exposure, not blistered.

The patient woke up and said, "I am waiting for the therapist."

"Everybody left already, come back tomorrow to continue with the therapy," the doctor said.

The patient reported feeling much better, but it was due to being placed in a face-down position more than from the light. The doctor felt it was the only good thing Sophia had accomplished.

After that day we reminded her to be more careful with patients. The incident made her drastically modify her procedure system.

Sometimes, with the pressure of time, paperwork, or distractions, anyone could inadvertently forget a patient in treatment.

CHAPTER TWELVE

Near-Death Experiences

W hether you believe in God or not, in health care services, you hear different stories about near-death situations from friends or read about them in books. But it is so different when you hear the stories first hand. Patients report experiences that make you think, and you come to understand they have a common denominator: peace.

A Surprise During Surgery

Mr. Gonzalez was a quiet and extremely gentle man, despite suffering severe back pain after surgery. He was always ready to flash his best smile. He was a very easy guy to talk to, and it was a pleasure to treat him. He was ready to cooperate during every session. Mr. Gonzalez was definitely a happy man.

After a few sessions treating him, I asked, "How could you be happy despite your pain after the back surgery?"

He answered by telling the most amazing story about his surgery. He was ready to come to the hospital and had arrived very early. The nurses prepared him for a very common surgery to take care of a herniated disc. He was comfortably waiting for the operation and was at the table when the anesthesiologist talked with him one last time.

The anesthesiologist told him, "Sweet dreams," and he didn't know anything else until the moment he woke up—during surgery. He said he woke up but was floating away from his body. He felt a great sensation of peace; he was at the top of the ceiling in the corner of the room. Mr. Gonzalez told me he was relaxed as he looked down at the staff and doctors, who gathered around the body below.

Then he realized it was *his* body! He saw one nurse take orders from the other doctors and another nurse drop something. Meanwhile, the other doctor almost tripped trying to get close to the patient on the table. Mr. Gonzalez heard a doctor, whose face was familiar, say, "We have to do something now or we'll lose him!" Then he watched as they brought the defibrillator to shock his heart. The doctor in charge very loudly announced, "Clear!" He saw the patient's body jump, then it seemed nothing happened and everybody began to run around again.

Suddenly, he said he became somewhat impatient and thought to himself, *That's my body! But how can I be floating away from it?* He started to panic. He wanted to go back to his body, but he couldn't. The fear came in waves, he said. He continued to watch what was happening below. Everybody was scurrying around, and the same doctor shouted again, "Clear!" The poor body jumped again, but this time Mr. Gonzalez said he felt his soul or spirit was pushed back *toward* his body—he felt it *through his head*, like a magnet.

He didn't know what else happened, but he woke up several days later with a severe pain in his back. He was anxious to tell everyone what happened to him. He was a bit lightheaded from the pain medications he was given, but Mr. Gonzalez was very clear about his near-death experience. He said knew he was dying and saw exactly what happened.

The doctor who came to visit him told him he had scared them that day. They couldn't understand why his heart suddenly acted differently then stopped. The doctor was also trying to tell him what was done to him.

Mr. Gonzalez looked at the doctor and said, "I know what happened to me, and I will describe it to you. I know because I was in the room watching it."

"First, you were in prone, face-down position," the doctor explained, "and second, you were under the influence of the anesthesia."

Mr. Gonzalez gave him a big smile and told the doctor he saw everything and described what he witnessed.

The nurse's assistant and the doctor listened to every detail. They couldn't believe what he had related and that it was completely correct. How did he know exactly what happened inside surgery? It was impossible; he was literally dead for several minutes. Mr. Gonzalez surprised everyone with his story, and his life changed dramatically afterward. He began to appreciate the importance of the simple things in life and live every day like it was his last.

He recovered quickly and was a joy to talk to or work with. After completing his therapy he gave a big hug to each one of us.

Mr. Gonzalez was an example of faith for us.

I remember his big smile and his spirit. One day he would feel that same peace again because he was no longer afraid to die.

A Car Accident

Mrs. Parker was a very successful businesswoman who drove her nice car on I-95 from Palm City south to West Palm Beach. If you have traveled in that area, you have noticed the area of Palm City is quiet, but going south after 4:00 PM it gets busy with trucks and people who commute.

Mrs. Parker was focused on getting to her next meeting via I-95 when suddenly a truck driven by a man who was under the influence of alcohol, crossed lanes and hit her car. Her car tumbled many times.

She saw a light then darkness. She was dead, she told me, but she felt an immense peace and a feeling so beautiful it was hard to describe.

She thought it was dark and was walking in a tunnel. She could feel her friends and relatives next to her, and they made her feel very comfortable. It was simply amazing, she said. She was so happy, then felt something pulling her back to life again.

She woke in the ER with severe neck pain. She had come back to life!

She later told me she was disappointed she had so much pain and was unable to move, but she was more upset with the doctors and nurses. Why had she been brought back to life only to suffer severe pain? It wasn't fair. She was literally ready to punch every doctor and nurse for that reason.

Not only could Mrs. Parker not move, she had some awful thing on her head and around her neck, shoulders, and chest. The nurse explained she had a halo device screwed into her skull to hold her neck in position until its broken vertebrae could heal.

Mrs. Parker was in shock.

After several weeks in the hospital and two months in rehab she was sent home, which was where I saw her for the first time. She had high hopes of accomplishing something positive in her treatment after having gone through so much torture. She didn't have the halo anymore and was cooperative with every session.

After I worked with her for several weeks at home, she wanted to come to the outpatient clinic therapy at our facility. We worked together several weeks, mainly to develop her skills in bed mobility and transfers. She couldn't walk due to paralysis in both legs; however, she was able to transfer using a sliding board from the wheelchair to the table. She managed to become quite independent and was very happy to have achieved her goal of mastering ample transfers skills. However, her life had changed dramatically since her accident, and she had to adapt to the paraplegia.

She told me about the peace and the happy feelings she experienced right after the other car impacted her car. She said, "I don't worry about death anymore, I just think one day my time will come, and I will be happy waiting for it. I know because of how I felt that day."

Both of these near-death experience stories have touched me. It doesn't matter how much book knowledge you've acquired, there is always a special feeling when you hear about experiences directly from the people who lived them. In each of these cases, someone described something similar, which was peace.

Some people give you other details, such as a light at the end of a tunnel or relatives waiting. It's not difficult for me to think that way because of my beliefs, but it is a comfort to hear stories like these because they give hope of a better tomorrow.

CHAPTER THIRTEEN

Beyond Manipulation

I was working in Houston, Texas as a young therapist, hoping to learn and work as much as possible to become a good, skilled professional in my field. I was the only one in my group who was bilingual (Spanish/English), which was quite strange for an area with such a large Hispanic population.

The hospital was located near a big oil refinery, and we received Workers' Compensation patients quite often. One day I worked with a young man, Ricardo, who had injured his left shoulder and developed the infamous "frozen" shoulder, a horrible stiffness and pain in the shoulder that creates difficulty in all activities of daily living.

I saw Ricardo because his English was quite limited; he was originally from Mexico. He was a very good patient who understood the shoulder had to be moved as much he could tolerate. The medicines didn't help much, so we had to use other modalities, such as heat, electrical stimulation, massage, and, mainly, manual therapy, which helps to move the joint and the soft tissue surrounding it. We worked for several weeks, but his progress was very minimal.

I went with Ricardo to his doctor's appointment, which was across the hall from our therapy department. I needed to both talk to the orthopedic physician and translate for my patient. The doctor agreed with me that Ricardo's improvements were very slow and said we should allow perhaps two more weeks of effort before putting him under anesthesia for manipulation, a technique used to actually break scar tissue while the patient is under anesthesia.

I was clear to my patient as I translated to him word for word what the doctor said. He understood that if nothing happened during his continued therapy, he would have to be admitted to the hospital for surgical manipulation so he would later be able to move his shoulder freely.

Ricardo's had not improved after two weeks, and the doctor scheduled the manipulation procedure. I accompanied Ricardo to the hospital and spent time to cheer him up. He was somewhat happy his shoulder was finally going to improve.

Ricardo was taken away to the anesthesiologist, who spoke Spanish, but I saw him again in the operating room. He was on the operating table with his left shoulder exposed.

The doctor greeted me and began a trivial conversation about the improvement of last weekend's football game, which was not uncommon for natives of Houston to do back then. Then he asked me which shoulder the patient had problems with.

I said, "The left one, doctor."

He asked me which movement was restricted.

I told him it was the external rotation, a backward movement, such as in baseball when a pitcher winds up to throw the ball.

The doctor then took Ricardo's left arm and was even more shocked at the restriction in its range of motion. He tried to move it but couldn't. Then he positioned himself and, using his whole body, performed the manipulation.

At that moment I heard the worst sound I had ever heard in my life; it sounded like the doctor was breaking a piece of wood—a horrible noise that had come from Ricardo's shoulder. I didn't know in what condition he was going to wake up after such an ordeal.

The orthopedic doctor asked me again, "Are there other problems with the shoulder?"

I remained quiet, because the damage was already done, and it seemed to me he was going to try something worse. I told him it was enough, and he left the room.

I stood there, shocked at the rough procedure just performed before my eyes. I had witnessed a similar procedure on someone's knees once, but the knees are much bigger and stronger joints. This was the first shoulder manipulation I had seen.

I stayed with Ricardo until he woke up, and, just as I had predicted, his pain was horrible. He screamed! The nurses didn't know what to do. The doctor was called and was reluctant to give him more medicine, but Ricardo was in terrible pain and they had already given him strong medication. Because it was an outpatient procedure, he was sent home that night.

Ricardo's pain was so severe that he couldn't sleep at all—for a week or more. The pain was bad for almost two months, but Ricardo received daily therapy, after which he regained very minimal range of motion. The biggest problems he still had were the swelling, bruises, and pain he experienced after the manipulation.

I have since learned a big lesson about the manipulation procedure for a frozen shoulder. I now understand I should try to avoid it and protect my patients from ever going through a similar experience. The outcomes and pain are so bad and negative that no patient should ever experience it. Ricardo took more than a year to recover from that episode. He could never use his shoulder again and ended up with disability because of his functional limitations.

The last time I saw Ricardo was before I left Texas, and his pain was minimal. He was finally able to perform the activities of daily living and drive his car, which was fitted with modifications.

Every time I have a similar case, I tell my patients Ricardo's story and conclude with this question: "Do you want to have a manipulation under anesthesia, or do you want to work hard with me and make progress? It will be a slow process, but it will happen."

CHAPTER FOURTEEN

My Friend, Bill

I worked in a small local hospital on the Treasure Coast of Florida, considered southeast Florida, and my position was the most important of my short career. At twenty-seven years of age I accepted the position to be in charge of starting an outpatient physical therapy business for the hospital. I saw the potential of the job and was excited to take it.

My staff consisted of one PT technician and a secretary. I had thirty patients on my first day, which is an impossible number for one person. With my assistant's help, we finished with our last patient at 7:00 PM.

The next day I called management and told them I needed help as soon as possible. They sent me a PT and a volunteer to help with tasks such as taking patients to the fitness center next door.

That was when I met Bill.

He was in his mid forties, tall, and thin. He had a cup of coffee in his hands, a big smile, and enthusiasm to work. I was impressed with the dedication he gave to each of the tasks assigned to him. I learned very quickly he was a wizard with computers and helped us tremendously when we couldn't solve our new computer system's problems.

Bill was from Nebraska and had owned a computer company there for years. He made a tremendous amount of money every month but one day decided to take his family—a wife and two kids—to Florida to pursue his dream of becoming a physical therapist. He sold his company and made a comfortable living off the sale.

He was very analytical and planned to finish his courses at the local college, to work volunteer hours, and to apply to one of south Florida's colleges. He was a very interesting person with many stories, most of which were hilarious. We became friends very quickly, and he often gave me good advice.

He invited me to eat one of his favorites foods, chicken wings, in the hospital cafeteria. I normally refused to eat there because, at the time, it had a bad reputation for giving diners stomachaches. One day, after he insisted, we went to the cafeteria to eat chicken wings, which was one of my worst culinary experiences. The wings were so spicy they burned my mouth for several hours and, of course, my stomach burned too. My friend Bill impressed me by putting more hot sauce on each chicken wing—and more salt. I had never seen anyone do that before; he pushed it to the limit.

Time passed and he still had not been accepted by the college. He received all kinds of excuses via mail: "You still need to complete an extra credit." In a very polite way they told him, "You are too old to apply to our school."

He never gave up and continued working toward his goal, waiting for any school to accept his application.

Unfortunately, his funds ran short, so I helped him to get a PT technician job to make a few bucks. It was difficult for a man who used to make a six-figure salary just a few years earlier.

At the same time, my personal life became a nightmare. After my son's birth, he had to be sent as an emergency patient to another hospital to have a quick but complicated abdominal surgery—with not much chance of survival.

My world came crashing down in pieces. I don't have close family here, so I felt alone, and I questioned my faith. I was devastated and couldn't think straight. At my lowest point I cried out of sheer frustration, away from my family because I didn't want them to see me that way.

It was then that my dear friend Bill came to see me. I didn't call him, he just found out and, without thinking, knew that his presence was important to me. I will never forget such a significant and beautiful gesture. He gave me a hug, and I couldn't stop crying. It felt as if I were hugging my father, which gave great comfort to my broken heart. Bill was the kind of friend you always want; he was there every step of the way for me, and I appreciated it so much.

My son's situation improved, and, when he finally came home, everything looked a little more normal, although he would have a long recovery.

A year or so after that, Bill called me late one night and gave me the best news: He was finally accepted by the college and was on his way to start his dream of becoming a physical therapist. He was like a little kid, so excited. (He separated from his wife due to their lifestyle change.) He was fifty years old when he started college for his new career. He went through all of the programs, and we called each other every weekend, making plans to start a new business together—maybe opening a PT clinic together—once he finished school.

One night when he was finishing his curriculum, I received the worst phone call. Bill was trying to tell me what was happening to him, but he was always joking, and this time was no different. Maybe he thought it would make it easier for me to digest the bad news to be joking around when he told me he had cancer of the esophagus. He said he would go for treatment the next week.

I was speechless. After all the years waiting for his dream, this was too much. I encouraged him to fight and never give up. He didn't want me to visit him after chemotherapy and radiation because his physical appearance was going to change so much. So I respected that and remained in touch by calling every day.

Bill managed to finish all of his programs and waited to take his licensure exam. We continued to make plans; we thought it was going to be possible for him to beat the disease.

But life had different plans for him.

One of his sons called me on a Monday night. The first thing I thought was that it couldn't be bad news because I had just talked to Bill on Saturday. But I was wrong. His son gave me the bad news: His father had passed away a couple of hours earlier. He was sick on Sunday and had to be hospitalized. He had gone into respiratory failure, was intubated, and depended on a ventilator to breathe until his death.

The news almost made me collapse. I couldn't believe it. My dear friend had died.

I went to Bill's funeral, and when it was my turn to speak, I could hardly talk. I just cried and cried. I tried to say how great his friendship had been, his encouragement, his perseverance to follow his dreams. Even though I am an experienced speaker, I just couldn't do it.

Bill left me something that you expect from a best friend who has died: First, the emptiness of his absence, and, second, the good memories that I was blessed to share with him.

CHAPTER FIFTEEN

Mr. Washington:
An Example of the Perfect Patient

I have always been connected to home health services during my career. For therapists, it is a good way to make extra money; besides,
it's a flexible schedule. Working with patients in their homes makes
each visit more interesting because you learn more about them and their
families, and, of course, you hear many stories.

A very common procedure for PTs is to check our schedule and
organize the day according to geographic area so we don't have to drive
more than necessary. That may be the worst part of working in the
physical therapy field: You drive and drive all day long, from patient to
patient. After a while, however, it's something you get used to.

It was a Saturday, approximately ten years ago, and not too many of
my colleagues worked on that day, but for me it was very normal. Maybe
by choice, but also because I have always carried a heavy case load. I
received a call to see Mr. Washington, who suffered from a vascular
problem in one of his legs. He had PAD (peripheral artery disease) and

underwent surgery in an attempt to fix the poor blood circulation in his lower legs. During the phone conversation to set up the appointment, he was very pleasant, and I thought it was good to have someone to treat who was nice.

The next day I was at his front door on time. I knocked and Mrs. Washington asked me to come in. I saw Mr. Washington sitting on the couch. He had a big smile, small eyes, and wore a baseball cap. He had quite a collection of caps embellished mostly with fishing or hunting decorations. He sat, ready to start his recovery at home for his swollen legs and feet.

His surgery was done in the groin to allow better circulation to his leg. He walked with difficulty with a walker from the family room to his bedroom, not more than twenty feet. He tried his best. He could handle a lot of work, and I was surprised by his enthusiasm. He demonstrated he wouldn't give up and was ready to fight any disease that came his way.

In some way my thought was prophetic: I feared Mr. Washington going back to the hospital. After a few weeks the vascular surgeon saw him and decided to do another surgery to attempt to save his legs, because the previous surgery had proved to be unsuccessful.

I was called again after the new surgery, and he was ready to work. This time was much easier because he knew me, and we laughed about different things. I used my strange sense of humor, and he loved it; Chilean humor is weird, and some people love it, especially Mr. Washington. He used to laugh so hard, I worried he would stop breathing.

Later, he again had to go for surgery. This time, his other leg presented the same problems and the pulses in his leg were slight to none. His doctor was worried; if he didn't act quickly, something serious was going to happen. Mr. Washington accepted the reality of everything happening to him, yet he still had a big smile and was ready for whatever would come his way. He wasn't worried at all—just ready.

After several years of spending more time in the hospital than home, and after so many surgeries, he lost one leg. I saw him many times during those years, but I never had the chance to complete any plan of care because he went to the hospital so often. By then we had established a good friendship, and he trusted my opinion and honesty about the situation.

The amputation was performed above the knee, and the wound was still healing. In addition, he also suffered congestive heart failure and leukemia. He had several volumes of medical records in the hospital, and everybody knew him because he was there so frequently, which is a sad way to have people know you. Doctors, nurses, technicians, they all knew him on sight.

Mr. Washington received chemotherapy at intervals and often went to the hospital due to severe weakness or other complications. It was hard to keep him at home with so many treatments and problems. However, we had managed to work some days in between the treatments.

Finally, there was a glimpse of peace and stability in his condition, and his heart was stable. His leukemia was also under control, and his new prosthesis from the VA hospital was finally ready, a new C-Leg. He worked hard to use it with a walker and with a cane for walking a few feet. He also loved the idea of being able to walk out of the house and move around without depending on anybody else, just his new C-Leg. Always happy and smiling, working hard, and never complaining, he was finally getting close to reaching his goals when, yet again, life pushed him back.

One day, his heart was not able to pump well and his leg became swollen. He fought it, but I had to convince him the edema in his leg was not normal and he needed to go to the ER. He didn't want to go, but after talking to him at length, he listened and trusted me. He went to the hospital with congestive heart failure, which was the beginning of the end. He couldn't go back to outpatient or walk with a cane. He became weaker and weaker, but his smile and happiness remained unchanged.

I used to ask him about his old job as a postal carrier. He was one of the first ones in this area and had many stories about dogs chasing him when he delivered mail.

His wife was always there. They made a beautiful couple and raised kids, grandkids, and great-grandkids. The weekends were busy for them because family members visited him frequently. On Saturdays when I went to see him, he always watched *The Three Stooges*. He loved those silly guys.

One Saturday I went to his house and saw his leg had swollen again with severe edema. I hated to tell him about it, but it was my job to inform him. I am a professional, but he was my friend too. I told him I was so sorry about the edema, but he had to go to the hospital immediately—it was an emergency. I could see a change of facial expression; it was the only time Mr. Washington revealed his sadness. But, being strong minded, he accepted it, and 911 was called due to his shortness of breath.

He never returned home. He knew it was the end; I think after all those years of fighting and fighting, he developed an intuition. He went downhill, but not without fighting. My staff and I were in constant communication with his family. Mr. Washington was in the hospital for a month when his body started to fail and couldn't tolerate any more treatments. He couldn't breathe by himself anymore; a respirator was the only thing keeping him alive.

I went to see him in the ICU. He was in critical condition yet could open his eyes from time to time. There was this man, lying in this hospital bed, connected to so many tubes. I extended my hand, and he squeezed it to show me his friendship. I noted his profound physical weakness in that simple gesture. Mr. Washington's eyes were open, and he tried to tell me something but couldn't talk because of his respirator tube. I understood he was saying, "Thank you!" It was beautiful, but I was shocked because he was always so tough and so happy. It was hard for me to see him that way and to say goodbye. His whole family was there too.

He was an inspiration for many people who complained about their life or pain. He was always ready to fight—with a big smile on his face. I don't believe I will have the pleasure to treat somebody like him again; he was unique. He was, simply, Mr. Washington.

CHAPTER SIXTEEN

Jimmy, My 6'8" Patient

J immy was a retired engineer who enjoyed living a quiet Florida lifestyle.

He had been diagnosed a short time earlier with Parkinson's disease but remained quite independent until tremors affected the use of his upper extremities. Jimmy and his wife researched until they found a doctor who specialized in surgical interventions that might control his tremors. Jimmy was better after the surgery and could perform his activities with less stress or difficulty.

One day he began to feel ill and was sent by emergency ambulance to the hospital. His brain had been affected by a blood clot, for which he underwent a crucial surgery. His wife knew he was going to endure a lot of recovery time if he was going to make it after surgery. He made it and was sent to a rehabilitation facility. He spent several weeks there and was later sent home with orders for home health care, which is how I met Jimmy.

My first day at his house, his wife opened the door. I met this wonderful lady with a very high spirit, always smiling, who told me she was ready to fight for Jimmy one more time. It didn't matter to her how much or how long it would take, she said she was ready to do it. And she remained next to her husband during every single step of his recovery. It inspired many of us to see real love in a couple together for so long.

Jimmy was very tall, 6 feet 8 inches, and required a special hospital bed; otherwise, his legs would stick out over the footboard. He was extremely weak and unable to move in bed or sit. He weakly moved his legs and stopped very frequently due to fatigue. Every session was tough for him, especially for a person who hated to do exercises. All his life, he didn't practice any sport. Being tall, he could have been great at basketball, volleyball, or any sport, but he only played chess. I couldn't believe it and teased him all the time, but Jimmy had a good sense of humor.

The first time his wife and I lifted him and placed him on his bedside in a seated position was really a daunting task. It was very difficult to keep him stable. His blood pressure dropped quickly, and he could faint at any time. We got him up to sit several times, and then the hard work finally paid off. He was able to sit with assistance at the edge of the bed and could eat his meals in a more natural position.

Later, he mastered maintaining the seated position so well that I tried to get him to stand. It would be the first time since his surgery, months earlier. We took all of the precautions possible; it was going to be the first time lifting him and checking how well he could hold a vertical position. We did that for three seconds, and Jimmy almost fainted, so I had to lay him down quickly.

We tried several sessions. Each time it was easier, and he helped more and more. Then he was ready to take his first few steps. It was a big deal for him, his wife, and for me, so we did it using a gait belt. He held my shoulders like a walker while his wife followed with the wheelchair. He took three steps and collapsed back into the chair. It wasn't pretty, but we did it.

I decided Jimmy was ready to try a walker adjusted to his height. He felt stronger, and we tried to walk outside in the street so he could be out and see all his neighbors, who were also very supportive. It was fun, and we did it for several months. Jimmy was a very quiet person but enjoyed being outside. He was able to move better and depend less on his wife, who worked so hard right along with him. Everything finally looked better. Then he started to develop urinary tract infections, for which he ended up in the hospital several times. Each time he became weaker and weaker. More work had to be done to emphasize his walking. He was unable to walk outside and needed a pacemaker to avoid fainting, which had happened quite often.

One day, right in a doorway, he took a few steps with me while his wife followed us with the wheelchair. He suddenly collapsed. Imagine a very tall person falling down directly to the floor. I broke his fall with the gait belt and held it very firmly, but his body was almost trapped between the door frame and the wheelchair. His wife was in the back and neither of us could go through the doorway; Jimmy was stuck there. I couldn't help his wife because I was worried about releasing the gait belt. If I let go of it, he could fall even lower and hurt himself. Seemingly out of nowhere, Jimmy's wife lifted him, and we put him back in the wheelchair. By then he was conscious again and asked what had happened.

After her show of strength, I told him, "Jimmy, don't upset your wife, otherwise she could beat the hell out of you!"

He laughed about that all the time.

He was continually sick with urinary tract infections, and each infection was worse. He was declining quickly and knew it. He didn't talk much and wasn't able to do much therapy. His wife was also dealing with her own health issues, but she was tough as an oak and continued taking care of him. She was an example to me of dedication and love.

Years earlier, Jimmy arranged with the Parkinson's Association and the University of Miami to donate his brain to research when he died, which always fascinated me. Jimmy was a practical man who wanted to give his body for research to help others, a very altruistic act that spoke volumes about his character.

The day he passed away finally came after he'd spent several long weeks in bed, unable to move. Once he was declared dead, his wife honored his wishes and followed the protocol requested by the University. She had placed ice bags around his body, especially his skull, to avoid any alterations for the future research.

I learned from Jimmy and his wife about love and support, as well as goals in life and how important it is to have somebody next to you who loves you unconditionally. Life twists and turns and changes things from one moment to another, but we have to be ready to give our best fight and never lose hope.

CHAPTER SEVENTEEN

The Cheerleader

I worked in Texas in the early nineties, and my job, like the rest of the staff, was constant rotation between inpatient to outpatient services. The hospital was a very good rotation because we were involved in the wound care program, which meant working with patients who had wounds or open sores unable to heal properly without intervention. We used whirlpools and were also in charge of cleaning, gentle debridement, and dressing each one of them.

I was there during my regular week when I received the referral of a seventeen-year-old girl, Christine, who was involved in a car accident with her boyfriend over the weekend. They drove in the fast lane late at night, irresponsibly, with a few drinks in their system, and in a Jeep without a roof cover. The combination of driving under the influence of alcohol, then suddenly having to stop because the car in front of them was going too slow for them, was not a good one.

The problem was, Christine wasn't wearing her seatbelt and flew forward with such force she broke through the windshield and ended up sliding in shorts across the pavement for seventy feet through the broken glass spread over the ground. The outcome of this incident made a horrible and painful combination for Christine. She felt the glass tear her skin, which was already burned from road rash. Pieces of her skin were gone in her knee area. She had raw skin on the fronts of her legs and on her side, but her pain also came from the large number of glass pieces embedded in both legs. It was a miracle she didn't have any fractures or other problems.

On Monday, when I started my rotation in the hospital, she was ready to start with therapy to allow for proper debridement to clean her wounds and begin the healing process. During her first treatment, a young doctor came to check on her, and we did the debridement together. The doctor and I explained the procedures to be done on her legs. Her mother accompanied her daughter to the first treatment using whirlpool to clean the wounds. Christine liked that part, even though the medicine in the water gave her a burning, itching sensation. But she got used to it quickly. What she hated with every fiber of her being was the next part: the cleaning and debridement. The skin on her legs had some black areas from the friction burn, bits of pavement were still attached to the skin, and multiple glass fragments remained.

I had never heard a young girl with such a bad "potty" mouth. She cursed and cursed every time I cleaned and debrided her wounds, but she made excellent progress. Her skin was healing and her knees were able to bend; however, I still found pieces of glass in her legs from time to time, which I used tweezers to remove. She screamed and swore again. I got used to the spectacle she created.

The family who came to be with her were completely shocked as they listened to her curse. It was unexpected because she looked so innocent and calm, but maybe it was her way to cope with the painful procedure. It took two months and several x-rays to be certain she didn't have a single piece of glass left in her legs. It wasn't until then she started to change and realize what she had gone through.

She left the hospital to live a normal life, but only after having learned an immense and important lesson: give thanks for the second chance.

She needed to change and become more responsible with herself. To this day, I hope she followed the right path.

Treating teen and young adult patients is always a challenge because their priority is basic: "Don't cause me pain during therapy." Unfortunately, most of the time there is only one way to proceed, and pain will be a result of the treatment. Physical therapists have to help them understand that, even though pain will be a factor, they will get better—and sooner rather than later—then they won't need further therapy and can enjoy life again.

CHAPTER EIGHTEEN

Driving Test

One of the ultimate skills physical therapists evaluate at home visits is the driving skill of a patient.

Mrs. Rowell was a ninety-one-year-old lady who had suffered a hip fracture that was repaired but required the implantation of hardware. She lived alone and went to rehab after her hospital stay.

Four weeks after she came home, I started her physical therapy. She was no more than four feet ten inches tall. I am six feet, one inch tall, so you can imagine how interesting we looked walking together in the street when we practiced her gait ability. Therapy was painful for her, but she tolerated it well. She wanted to get back to her regular routine, so she worked hard to get her strength and balance back.

Mrs. Rowell always wanted to walk close to her car as part of her training and therapy. I could see her eyes widen and a look of satisfaction come across her face every time she saw her car. She asked me over and over, "When I can drive my car?"

Each time, I explained to her, "You have to be able to walk steadily, improve your strength and balance, then you will be able to get in and out of the car, and move your right hip."

Normally, when it is the right hip, there is a more conservative approach to therapy to make sure the patient demonstrates the strength and appropriate reactions for driving. I told Mrs. Rowell the next time she saw her orthopedic doctor, I was going to send a letter to ask him about her driving. I knew the doctor and thought he would also tell her she needed to be a little bit patient. Then we waited.

More therapy continued, and she was really showing progress. Before, she'd had pain just from sitting or standing from the chair, but now the pain was gone. Mrs. Rowell had been very unsteady with her first couple of steps with a walker but was now able to get up using a cane, and she did so very steadily. I was impressed with her vitality and her willpower. Patients like her made me feel good about my work and motivated me. PTs always hope to have patients like Mrs. Rowell.

Finally, she went to see her doctor, who was also impressed with her recovery. She was very anxious to ask him about driving. He said yes to driving, but I was to be the one to take her for a test drive to judge her skills.

I went to see her the next day, which was her last session with me at her home.

Mrs. Rowell waited for me with a big smile and wide eyes. Finally, she was going to drive after three long months! She had hated not driving because she'd depended on so many people for her transportation. Besides, she loved her big car. She was ready, and I told her we were going to review some of the therapeutic exercises first, check a few things, then do the driving test.

I was nervous, like I said, because I didn't know how good her driving skills were.

The moment of truth came. Mrs. Rowell took her car keys and purse, and we walked to her car parked in the driveway. She opened the door and got in, and I entered the passenger's side. We both put on our seatbelts. She adjusted the rear view mirror then started the car. Her excitement was obvious, but she backed up the car very slowly.

Then came one of the most nervous times in my life. Mrs. Rowell started to drive—like a maniac! She was transformed, not the same lady I knew. The look in her eyes scared me, and she drove very fast. She was speeding, and the worst part was the curves.

My God, but she was in ecstasy!

It came to a point when I was so nervous I asked Mrs. Rowell, "Can you slow down please? I am very nervous with your driving!"

"Don't worry, honey," she said to me, "I've been driving this way all my life."

This is crazy! I thought. I begged her to go back to her house.

Mrs. Rowell listened to me, but then came the worst part. When we arrived at her home, she needed to park her car in a very tight garage. And she didn't slow down!

I thought I was going to be in the obituary section of tomorrow's newspaper, captioned, "PT Dies in the Hands of Crazy Lady!" She drove like a maniac! Seriously, I have never been so scared in my entire life. I have tested many patients' driving skills, taking into consideration the skills necessary to get in and out the car, and other components related to therapy, but that time was something I won't forget.

Mrs. Rowell parked the car like in the movies, at high speed, yet so perfectly.

When she stopped the motor, my heart was still beating fast. I asked her, "Do you seriously drive like that all of the time?"

She said, "Yes!" Then she told me she hadn't ever had a ticket or an accident, which I thought was a miracle.

I expressed my concerns, but at the same time I asked her to call me every time she got in her car or to put a big red flag on her car next time she was driving around so it would be easy for me to recognize her. I left her that day with my legs still shaking and thanking God for keeping us unharmed.

The goal to work in the field of rehabilitation is to return functional skills to the patient. Sometimes we have to directly test our results, and surprises like Mrs. Rowell can bring us a very happy—or stress-inducing—memory.

CHAPTER NINETEEN

The Difficult Patient

P hysical therapists, like any other health care professionals, go through the same procedure, day after day, of checking our schedules to see how many and which patients we will have. Sometimes we hold our head with both hands as a reaction when we learn a particular patient is scheduled. Some patients can be quite difficult, and we wonder how tough their appointment will be that day.

Years ago I went to see the most difficult patient to whom I had ever been exposed: Mr. Weber. From time to time, all of us meet people who are not too nice or are a real pain in the neck, but this patient was by far the worst for me.

Physical therapists always receive referrals. I accepted his and planned to call him to arrange a visit for the next day. It is the regular procedure I have followed for years. I call all of my patients the night before I visit them to ask if everything is okay with them and to be sure it won't be an inconvenience for me to be there. I work to avoid conflicts with doctors' appointments and family situations.

I made the phone call, and Mr. Weber answered with "Call me later, I am eating my dinner."

I understood and called him forty-five minutes later.

He answered and asked, "Why are you calling me this late?"

Then I said, "I did call earlier, but you were eating dinner."

Mr. Weber didn't like that; he said I should have called him five minutes after the first call, even though he told me to wait forty-five minutes. Then he started to question my background, so I explained to him about my qualifications and experience in the field.

Mr. Weber asked if I was familiar with the surgical procedures performed by his orthopedic doctor.

I replied saying I was very familiar with the procedures and had worked with many patients with the same diagnosis who had been referred by the same doctor.

He wasn't pleased with my explanation and asked me who referred him to me.

Again, I tried to explain him how the referral procedure worked, but he didn't care much at all. I told him I would like to arrive mid-morning, but he got upset because *he* wanted to pick the time for me to be there. I explained to Mr. Weber we could compromise if he had a problem with that particular time, but his excuse was he needed that specific time for coffee and to read the newspaper. I told him he wasn't my only patient and the time I had chosen was the best time.

Suddenly, he began yell at me. He was literally screaming at me from the other side of the phone.

I gently told him he needed to calm down before I could continue talking.

Mr. Weber kept yelling at me then hung up the phone.

I called him again to attempt to clear up the situation, but his reaction was the same. I began to lose *my* cool and raised *my* voice. My family was worried that I was yelling too; I normally do not have that type of reaction, especially with patients. I was so upset with Mr. Weber. I only wanted to help him to recover from his surgery.

"Fine, come over around ten," Mr. Weber said.

We finally agreed.

I was curious and also not too excited to see Mr. Weber, but I am a professional and accepted him in my case load because I knew he needed my services. I rang the door bell, and a man started yelling, "I'll be there!"

I gave him enough time to get to the door and waited as long as necessary.

Then he opened the door and gave me a creepy smile.

I introduced myself and explained why I was there. After talking and talking, I realized Mr. Weber suffered from a lot of pain. It turned out his pain medications weren't working, and he wasn't taking them properly.

I gave him my suggestions, and he listened to me for the first time. I performed my evaluation and treatment, and left.

The next day, Mr. Weber was very nice to me and thanked me because he had a decent night, which was the breaking point of his nastiness.

At every following session he was more open, and we talked like good friends. He was happy to see me and allowed me to help him work with the therapeutic exercises for his leg.

After time, Mr. Weber showed me how nice he was, which I thought was a huge transformation. I was happy with the outcome. He was able to walk without a walker and with less pain; he was clearly recovering.

The last day of therapy came, and he wanted to continue. I told him my office was on the other side of town, about thirty minutes away, compared to other ones only five minutes away. He insisted, and I saw him at my office. He came to every session and was the most fun, kind patient in the whole case load. I couldn't believe the transformation!

I told him I learned something from him: First impressions are not always accurate. I also learned pain and lack of sleep can make a person act nasty as hell.

I felt a great feeling of accomplishment after that experience. It demonstrated that my profession can help patients reach not only physical goals but mental ones as well.

CHAPTER TWENTY

Travel to Jordan

M rs. Quinn had just moved to Florida from New York, where she had lived most of her life. She was very happy in her marriage of more than thirty years, but her husband had died of a lung disease, which took much out of her and the whole family. She decided to continue with the plans her husband had made before his death and move to the house they had bought in Florida.

She was devastated at being alone, but she knew she had to go. It was a tough decision, but her family understood. She finally moved to her new house and was just starting to settle in when her right hip started to hurt. Each day, due to the activity of moving to the new house, she experienced severe pain in her groin.

She went to see a doctor, who right away referred her to an orthopedic physician. The orthopedic doctor took an x-ray and could see she needed a new hip as soon as possible.

She thought about it and agreed; she couldn't carry on with the current pain or limitations. She also knew it was going to be difficult and severely painful, but she was ready.

During that time she had a very peculiar dream of being in a different but very old town, perhaps from centuries ago, where she saw herself as happy and at peace, with kids surrounding her. The dream repeated more frequently. She was worried and told her family, some of whom were in town to help her after the surgery and with the unpacking.

Her surgery was completed successfully, and she was recovering at home when she was referred to me.

I recognized the address as a house I had been in with another patient just six months earlier. I always felt something special in that house, maybe something more spiritual to me, something that made me want to go back because I felt a great deal of tranquility and peace there. It is difficult to explain. Maybe it was the way the distribution of the rooms allowed the light to stream into every corner, a nice view, and access to the backyard was open and featured a variety of beautiful and colorful flowers.

But there was something else in that house I understood later when I met Mrs. Quinn. I could see a tough and optimistic lady who, even though the circumstances had put her through a test, was able to keep going because of her constant hope. She learned to cope with her husband's death with more clarity after all the devastation and sadness she endured just a few months earlier. Now Mrs. Quinn was settled in the new house, with members of her family temporarily helping her, and recovering from surgery for a new hip.

She was a very good patient who did everything I requested during her therapy. She was also very disciplined and quite interested in spiritual things.

I mentioned to Mrs. Quinn about what this house made me feel, and she agreed with me. I said, "Good, so I am not crazy."

She told me about her dream, the one in which she saw herself in a town square surrounded by children. She said she'd told her family a decision she'd made: Once she got better, she was going to travel to Jordan. She told me her whole family said it was "too far," or "crazy," or she had "no business being there." But Mrs. Quinn insisted she was going to go to Jordan once she recovered, and that was that.

She finished her therapy "with honors," as we say in physical therapy when the patient does excellent work and always follows the program established. She had done well, and nobody could make her change her mind. She was going to Jordan. She bought her plane ticket and went on her own. She didn't allow any of her family members to go with her; she needed to do this alone. She described a strong force inside her that drove her to travel to Jordan.

After the trip, I had the chance to talk to Mrs. Quinn. I was curious, but I expected she'd had a great trip.

She told me that, when she arrived in Jordan, she was taken by a taxi to the hotel where she changed clothes and left for a walk. She somehow she knew exactly where to go. Mrs. Quinn couldn't believe it, but she walked those streets as if she had lived there for many years. It was so strange, she said she walked directly to the town square with a water fountain. She sat next to it and closed her eyes to enjoy the breeze and the people walking. In her mind's eye she saw herself in a white tunic dress playing with kids; she was a teacher.

Finally, she understood her dream and felt peace like never before. After many months of sadness, she finally felt the peace she sought. Her heart had been lifted up. She understood she had been there—in another life.

Many things made Mrs. Quinn believe it. Not only her dream, but she also couldn't explain how she could walk those streets without guidance, how she could understand the language, and those visions that made her so happy. They turned out to be the best treatment for her soul.

I never saw her again, but Mrs. Quinn's story made me think she was blessed to have a chance to find peace and happiness after her husband's death. I see so many widows or widowers who cannot recover from the loss and lose the purpose of their life. They just survive, waiting for their time, when instead they should be living without waiting.

CHAPTER TWENTY-ONE

Mary, the PT Technician

I have had many PT techs work with me through the years and, co-incidentally, with two technicians named Mary. It almost seems as if their name made them have similar personalities. They were always joking, had positive attitudes, were a pain in the neck at times, and they unexpectedly surprised us all the time.

In the physical therapy department, we always support each other. I suppose it's because we work so closely with patients and establish warm relationships. As a result, we are always celebrating something—birthdays, the last session of a particular patient, a holiday.

The clinic where I once worked was under renovation, so for about a month we all had to share a sink to wash our hands. One day, a patient brought us Italian food, including a salad, as a way to say thank you. We didn't have paper plates, but we had regular plates we used before the renovation—a gift from another patient the year before. Nobody thought about anything other than eating, so we did. Mary was the one in charge, like a mother who takes care of her kids. She was older than me and several of the others. We had a good lunch to celebrate.

When we finished, the plates had to be cleaned, so Mary said, "Don't worry, I'll take care of them" and left. We thought she took them to another area of the building where she could clean them, but she came back very quickly with the plates clean as new. Everyone was shocked and didn't ask her any details.

We returned to work with the patients on the afternoon shift. I was scheduled for a patient who needed the whirlpool treatment for her foot. She was recovering from an ankle fracture and had a small open sore area, so whirlpool treatment was perfect for her. I followed procedure and, while the patient was in the waiting room, prepared the whirlpool, filling it with water and adding a specific medicine.

After only a few minutes, the whirlpool was filled with warm water. I started the motor and everything was quite normal to disperse the medicine. Suddenly, I saw something strange thing float by. Was it a piece of lettuce? I wasn't sure. I thought maybe something was wrong with the machine, so I stopped it and called for one of my colleagues.

She came and offered the same opinion: A piece of lettuce floated in what was supposed to be sterile water.

The conclusion was quite easy: Mary had cleaned the dishes in the whirlpool! It was disgusting and very dangerous for patients.

How could I possibly approach her about it? Something definitely had to be done. I talked to her right away and told her what she had done was highly inappropriate. She needed to be cautious for the patients' safety as well as our safety.

I told her I understood we were renovating the clinic, but she still had to use common sense. She sterilized the whole whirlpool area. I made her do it twice, just in case.

I talked to the patient outside and told her we had some technical problems, but the treatment would begin shortly.

I don't remember any other incident like that one. It seemed Mary learned her lesson, and we did too. We used paper plates from then on.

CHAPTER TWENTY-TWO

The Wild and Brilliant Idea

I received a call from a recruiter to work in a local hospital to develop its outpatient therapy department. As I mentioned earlier, it was a professional challenge in which I saw potential. Years later, the outpatient therapy grew the way I suspected, which confirmed my sixth sense about it.

In the beginning, we had so many patients to work with that we had everything—except room. My staff and I pushed administration to commission the blueprints to renovate, improve, and increase the treatment rooms. But we needed to get someone from the board of directors to see the predicament and approve the improvements. I arranged for the director of rehab to help me.

The person scheduled to come was Mrs. Thompson, a very tough lady who had been very involved with the hospital for many years. But she was extremely conservative. We tried to make her understand how important the renovation was, but she was hard of hearing. "Selective hearing loss" might have been a better way to have described it.

We asked Mrs. Thompson to visit the PT department on our busiest day, Monday, which was also a busy day for the entire hospital. We didn't know what time she would arrive, but one of her secretaries, a previous patient of ours, planned to let us know when she was coming.

Perfect, but my PT tech Mary wasn't convinced about the value of the visit and told me Mrs. Thompson wouldn't do anything about our renovation. Mary said she'd planned something else to make the point about our need for rennovation.

It was busy when we received a call from the secretary, who told us Mrs. Thompson was coming at 11:00 AM. She was always punctual, so we were ready.

But Mary was already brewing her plan. She told me she had an idea. "Let's put two people on the big table with hot packs," she said, "one facing north the other facing south."

I wasn't sure, but I thought it might work. I knew Mary had been an employee at the hospital for many years, so she knew the staff well.

One patient was a black man with a knee problem, and the other was a blonde lady with shoulder pain. I told them our tricky plan, and they agreed to help us. They were extremely nice and knew how much we were pushing to get our clinic expansion.

Everything was ready when Mrs. Thompson came. I gave her a quick tour of the clinic, which was very small. Then came the grand finale. She came to the treatment room, and I still remember her face. Her eyes were wide open, almost like in a cartoon, and her jaw dropped.

Everyone was very tense, except for Mary, who was about to burst into tears of laughter.

I didn't know what to say, except, "Well, Mrs. Thompson, I hope you understand what I have been trying to tell you for several months. We really need more rooms and space."

Before I could continue she asked, "But what is this? You have people sharing the tables?"

I explained to her we didn't have any space, but the patients were okay with it.

She gave me a strange look. I couldn't read her expression, because her blank expression didn't reveal whether she was mad, shocked, or sad. She had a complete poker face.

"Okay," she finally said. "I will call the members to have an extraordinary meeting this afternoon to start working on the plan of expansion," and she left.

Two minutes later, I received phone calls from the administration office, including from the CEO, which was crazy.

I couldn't believe it. I told Mary she was right. I thought, from the tense situation, we were going to be in big trouble; instead, it was an amazing outcome.

Mary was right, she knew the people in the hospital community. Even though it was a big gamble, because of Mary we were able to have a more decent and bigger place for our patients.

Some of the most crazy ideas end up being the greatest ideas, like Mary's. I thanked her for her work, as I always do with all the people who work with me or for me. It is essential to show respect and leadership and to listen carefully to all kinds of ideas.

CHAPTER TWENTY-THREE

The 350-Pound Patient with Bilateral Knee Replacements

I was practically a new graduate when I went to work in a small hospital on the west coast of Florida. I was prepared for new challenges and learning. In those days, knee and hip replacements were the most frequent surgeries done at that hospital because they had two groups of orthopedic doctors. There was almost a competition between them to see which group could treat more patients than the other.

John, a retired merchant marine, was six feet, six inches tall and 350 pounds. He suffered with severe pain and stiffness in his knees, and decided to go for surgery. The doctors in one group offered to do both knees at the same time, a very new procedure for that hospital. Everybody was excited—except the staff in the physical therapy department.

Because John was very tall and heavy, he required both a special bed and walker. He was ready for everything except the pain.

The surgery was performed, and the doctor wanted to start with therapy right away. I received the order and took my assistant to help me because John's case was well known in the whole hospital for a couple of weeks.

I walked into the room and saw a very tall man lying over the bed, both knees wrapped in plenty of bandages. He was in pain and not happy to receive therapy. He refused to get up because the pain doubled when he tried. My assistant and I helped him with some range of motion exercises, but we left with an understanding that we would return in the afternoon, at which time he *would* get up on his feet.

The afternoon came, but John didn't change his attitude.

This time, I insisted he needed to get up, but all I could accomplish was to get him to sit at the edge of the bed and put his feet on the floor. He felt too much pain to do anything else and wanted only to lie in bed again.

The next morning, as he was doing his rounds, I explained to the orthopedic doctor how John refused to get up and walk. The doctor went to talk to John, and this time John was motivated to get up by a lecture from the doctor about blood clots and poor healing.

John agreed to give it another try.

Great! I thought, *It's a big change from yesterday.*

My assistant and I sat John at the edge of the bed and explained that, while he was going to have to stand, we were going to help him. One of us was positioned on each side of him, and with a gait belt we tried and tried to help him stand. He didn't cooperate much, and he was too big a load for just the two of us to lift. We tried later but were again unsuccessful.

The orthopedic doctor was unhappy with John and told me, "You have to find a way to get him up."

I came back to lift John safely with a team of five of the strongest therapists available—all prepared to accomplish the task.

John saw my big crew walk into the room and knew it was the day he was going to stand up and take a few steps, whether he wanted to or not. I was to be positioned at his back, so I had to climb in his bed, planning to push him from there. Two therapists stood by each of John's sides, and the fourth held the walker in front and tried to pull him from there. The fifth stood and acted as a cheerleader while waiting to see if his help was needed.

Everyone was in position, and because he was my patient, I gave the orders.

I announced, "Okay, on the count of three, we pull him up. One, two, and three!"

All of us lifted at once, and John quickly found himself standing.

The entire nursing staff on that floor heard a loud scream and ran into the room. They thought something bad happened but were surprised when they saw this big, tall guy standing with four therapists holding him. Everybody applauded. It really took a team effort, and I thanked my colleagues.

The first two or three steps John needed to take on his own. He took the first step, which led to another. It was getting a little dangerous; I noticed he was sweating profusely and thought it might be his blood pressure. He took another step and he said he felt faint, so we quickly put him back in bed.

All of us were sweating along with him.

After that day, John began to walk more and more. In four days he was walking with the walker—with supervision—around the nursing station and down the halls on that floor.

When John finally left the hospital, he had a special feeling of accomplishment. We were just as happy as he was.

From time to time, physical therapists have challenges due to patients' complexities, and a common challenge is a physical one. I have seen big patients working with short therapists or obese patients working with very thin ones. We have to learn to adapt to such diversity for both patient and therapist safety. But sometimes we have to be creative to help a patient take that first step, which is always the most difficult. I have found brainstorming with colleagues is always the best way to achieve success when challenges arise.

EPILOGUE

Life is full of stories and situations that make us understand why we experience both sweet moments as well as sour ones, a perfect roller-coaster. Sometimes we live believing we are in the middle of a dark night with almost no hope. Then we see a beautiful sunrise, the sun illuminates our path in life, and we recover from the sadness.

Recounting every one of these physical therapy stories makes me understand that I have been blessed. First and foremost, I'm blessed to be alive and able to remember each one of them. In my profession I have seen so many terrible situations and difficult diagnoses. People feel hope in physical therapy professionals and a chance to relieve their pain, or remove a physical limitation, or improve functional skills.

I have used the "fall" stories to forewarn my patients about the possibility of a fall, and they listen very carefully. Sometimes, in moments of pain, I tell them the funny stories to divert their attention.

If you can relate to one or more of the stories, it's because you've heard about something similar somewhere, or you went through it yourself, or a family member had a similar experience.

I continue to collect more stories, day by day; something new is always happening. In the meantime, I continue to educate and instruct my patients in the best ways to keep themselves safe so they can hold hope for a new sunrise.

APPENDIX A

How to Find a Physical Therapist

The public can learn more about the roles of a physical therapist, and physical therpaist assistants, by visiting the Federation of State Boards of Physical Therapy's website http://www.fsbpt.org/ThePublic/Learn-PhysicalTherapyBasics.aspx. Described on that page:

- Why one should seek a licensed practitioner
- Understand what physical therapists do
- Understand what physical therapy assistants do
- Learn about the types of treatments
- Discover areas of specialization
- Find out where PTs and PTAs practice

To find a licensed physical therapist in your area, first contact your health insurance provider for a list of approved providers. If you are uninsured or wish to connect with an out-of-network provider, choose "Find a PT" at the American Physical Therapy Association's website for patients: http://www.MoveForwardPT.com/Default.aspx.

Guidelines on how to select a physical therapist can be found at http://www.moveforwardpt.com/Resources/Choose.aspx.

APPENDIX B

How to Become a Physical Therapy Professional

Doctor of Physical Therapy

A Doctor of Physical Therapy (DPT) program is the degree course a prospective physical therapist will pursue. (The Master of Physical Therapy (MPT) and Master of Science in Physical Therapy (MSPT) degrees are no longer offered to new US students.) A DPT student learns theory, examination and evaluation, diagnosis, prognosis, treatment intervention, prevention, and consultation.

To practice as a physical therapist in the US, a student must earn a physical therapist degree from a physical therapist education program accredited by the Commission on Accreditation in Physical Therapy Education- (CAPTE-) accredited. A list of accredited schools can be found at http://www.capteonline.org/Programs/. CAPTE is the only accreditation agency recognized by the United States Department of Education (USDE) and the Council for Higher Education Accreditation (CHEA) to accredit entry-level physical therapist and physical therapist assistant education programs. According to its website, "CAPTE currently accredits over 200+ physical therapist education programs and over 250 physical therapist assistant education programs in the US and three physical therapist education programs in other countries . . ."

After school, the DPT student must then pass:

1. *the national physical therapy exam*, through the Federation of State Boards of Physical Therapy Examinations (FSBPT) at http://www.fsbpt.org/ExamCandidates/NationalExam(NPTE).aspx. FSBPTA is a membership organization with a mission to improve protect the public in 53 jurisdictions by providing service and leadership that promote safe and competent physical therapy practice.

2. *a state licensure exam.* A list with links to state licensing authorities' names, emails, phone and fax numbers and websites can be found at http://www.fsbpt.org/FreeResources/LicensingAuthoritiesContactInformation.aspx

3. and, in some states, students must also take *a jurisprudence exam*, which covers the practice act and rules under which licensed individuals are allowed to work.

Physical Therapy Assistant

A Physical Therapy Assistant (PTA) works under the direction and supervision of a DPT. The degree course a prospective physical therapy assistant will pursue is an associate degree from an accredited PTA program (two years, usually five semesters) at a technical or community college, college, or university. PTA program graduates must pass a national examination for licensing, certification and regulation in most states to be eligible to work.

To learn more about becoming a physical therapy professional, prospective DPT and PTA students can research "Careers and Education" at the American Physical Therapy Association (APTA) website: http://www.apta.org/. APTA is a membership organization of more than 90,000 physical therapists (PTs), physical therapist assistants (PTAs) and students. Its mission, according to its site, is "to improve the health and quality of life of individuals in society by advancing physical therapist practice, education and research, and by increasing the awareness and understanding of physical therapy's role in the nation's health care system."

ABOUT THE AUTHOR

Fernando Figueroa is the owner of Fernando PT Services in Stuart, Florida. He earned a bachelor of science degree in kinesiology in 1987 from the Univeristy of Antofagasta in his native Chile and his master's of science degree from Barry University in Miami, Florida in 1995. In 1999 he received a Ph.D. in health services administration from Columbia Southern University in Alabama and in 2007 his Doctor of Physical Therapy from the University of St. Augustine, Florida.

Dr. Figueroa is certified as an ergonomic evaluator specialist, Certified McKenzie-MDT. He also volunteers as a clinical instructor for physical therapist assistant students at nearby Indian River State College.

He has two children, a grown daughter and son. He enjoys tennis, running, playing chess, writing, riding his motorcycle, and sailing.

CPSIA information can be obtained
at www.ICGtesting.com
Printed in the USA
FFOW02n1327140317
33487FF